PATANJALI'S YOGA PHILOSOPHY

Author Page

How many times have you had to give up on a lifelong dream just because you thought you did not have the resources or skills needed to achieve them? How often do you let your circumstances define what your short- and long-term future will turn out to be? If you are like any other individual, chances are that you may be hiding your greatest dream and desires in the back of the last drawer, never to see the light of day.

I used to be like this, living with a passive attitude, letting the tides of life shape my present, and what was to become of me. I worked a 9 to 5 job at a bank for the longest time, doing the same thing over and over again and being able to learn and grow in the marketing field. But something deep inside me always knew that I could be doing so much more- so much more of what my heart has always wanted to achieve.

So, I took the chance, put on my hiking boots, and prepared to straddle the hills of struggle no matter what it took. Thirteen years later, I have finally conquered my fears and doubts and am ready to share my experience of immersing myself in the world of business development and entrepreneurship with young professionals like me who just need that little bit of a nudge of motivation to get them going.

I am Dr. Sriram Ananthan from Canada, and I am an entrepreneur, coach, leader, speaker, writer, yogi and, most importantly, a friend. What I aim to do with my knowledge and experience is to channel it all towards creating a well-rounded experience for anyone who needs guidance to get their professional lives on track.

Table of Contents

INTRODUCTION TO YOGA AND ITS LINEAGE

The precise root of yoga is still a mystery. There is some evidence to indicate that early forms of yoga may have occurred as far back as 2500-1500 BCE in the Indus Valley region of India. Sculptures of figures sitting in what looks like lotus postures have been found from this period, but since the script that accompanies the figures is unclear, it is not possible to say with any certainty if the sculptures are depictions of a yoga pose, or simply a way of sitting on the floor.

What is obvious is that from the earliest times there has been an awareness that human consciousness is immense, that it can be explored and from this discovery, discoveries emerge as revealed knowledge about the human existence, the world and our place in it. In India in the early centuries of the first millennium BCE two types of culture existed: Vedic, and non-Vedic.

The Vedas had sacred texts of revealed knowledge, or Sruti, meaning "that which is learned from a higher source." The four Vedas are the oldest scriptural text of the Hindu religion. The non-Vedic Indian community included Jainism and Buddhism, neither of which acknowledged the authority of the Vedas and thus developed into separate religions. It is important to note that, within the Indian community, wisdom was conveyed orally from Guru to the student: the Guru weaving threads of his wisdom into something meaningful and appropriate for that student. Owing to this form of transmission of knowledge, various philosophical schools have interacted and shaped each other in a much less linear manner than we would expect. It's uncertain if the yoga originated from Vedic or non-Vedic culture. Scholars have noted that Sramanas (literally, "those who exert themselves") was involved in austerities during this period — activities performed by renounced individuals and ascetics from non-Vedic culture.

Established tradition: Upanishad, Buddhism, and Jainism. The Bhagavad Gita was written shortly after the fifth century and was possibly completed before the end of the millennium. Within the sacred Indian text, there is nothing short of a revolution in Yogic philosophy. Yoga practice is growing. Different modes of practice are described: karma yoga, or the yoga of action; bhakti-yoga, or the yoga of devotion; and jnana yoga, or the yoga of research and awareness. In this way, all are made open to the practice of yoga and the highest states of consciousness, and it is not appropriate to renounce the universe and retreat into a cave. The text also suggests women are not exempt from this activity, a first in the history of yoga.

A brief overview of Patanjali, the founder of Yoga

Patanjali was a great Ancient India scholar. Some claim that he existed before Christ and some a little after Christ. We also don't know his exact dates. To discipline his vocabulary, he wrote a book on grammar. A second monumental medical work that will help us look after the body. Finally, he wrote a masterpiece in 195 short sentences or other aphorisms to teach us how to manage the mind, the Yoga Sutra.

It's said there would have been a loss today without Patanjali Yoga. "If you can't understand Patanjali, you're not going to understand Yoga, not with all the comparable literature on Yoga." The Yoga Sutra is not a practice manual for Yoga. It deals with the theory of yoga and the student, but means and methods for all types of students, from beginner to ready. So ask your yoga instructor, first of all, to tell you about the work of Patanjali! Here you can find a brief explanation of the first sutra, which is the answer to the question: what is trully yoga and why do we need to use techniques?

The 3 components of matter, namely Sattwa (purity, harmony, lucidity), Rajas (energy, passion) and Tamas (inertia and darkness), form the mind, according to Samkhya philosophy, on which the Yoga Sutra is grafted. They are responsible, negative or positive, for all of the mental changes or behaviors. For eg, it means being responsible for the distractions and limitations when Sattwa is just not enough in our personalities and Tamas is too much. Usually we listen rather than the light to the dark side within of us.

They are The Ego's three constituents. On Monday we feel clear-minded and concentrated, full of energy, but on Thursday we feel exhausted and frustrated because of all the energy that was used the day before and no target can appear any more clearly ... This state of mind has been witnessed by us, all of us. The consequences of the mental changes are these emotions, this instability. For the person, they may become very heavy and cause chronic depression, chronic tiredness, before the mental disorder. Patanjali here offers a sincere Yoga practice to stop this eternal process, to get out of misery. Therefore yoga is the regulation of mental shifts. By training, our minds grow healthier.

THE ORIGINAL PURPOSE OF YOGA

Below are some of the benefits of yoga that address the question 'why should you do yoga?

1. It overcomes tension

In this world tension is foreign to everyone.Often we all get upset and dissatisfied with life. And we get nervous. For most people managing stress is extremely difficult, which leads to long-term stress accumulation. Accumulation of stress normally causes an imbalance in your nervous system which makes it difficult for you to concentrate, sleep, and unwind. Promoting relaxation also helps the body lower the stress hormone cortisol. This will ease you more, and enhance your quality of life.

2. Helps to treat diabetes

If you are at high risk for diabetes, you will be glad to know that yoga will help you to reduce and control your diabetes risk. How? Yoga helps you fight diabetes by reducing the contributing factors which lead to diabetes. When you practice yoga, you generally do postures, which move back and forth between poses. Some of these poses contract those areas of your abdomen while others loosen certain areas.

3. It helps to improve immunity

Practising yoga lets you move through your organs continuously as you contract and stretch your muscles.

Usually, when you do so you increase the drainage of lymph in your body. Lymph is a viscous fluid rich in immune cells; thus, it enhances your immune defences as it is more widely dispersed across the body, increasing the body's immunity to internal and external attacks.

4. It makes you happy

One of the reasons why we feel depressed and angry as human beings are that we are not living in this moment.Let me break it down for you; most people spend time focusing on the past or the future. It keeps us occupied with preparation, worrying or regretting what it is doing to us. All this just heightens our nervousness and makes us feel helpless. Practice Yoga typically helps you to meditate. Meditation helps unplug your emotions and lets you reflect on what's happening in your body and your life. This is where happiness makes its way into the present.

5. Enhance Versatility

You can do yoga for one reason so that you can improve your flexibility.Yoga is usually full of postures that will work the whole body and include even the forgotten joints. This makes for a strong sense of balance and harmony. When you practice yoga, the muscle groups start working together instead of working against each other; and that is what makes you versatile. In the beginning, you can not feel this versatility, but if you stick to it, you will be shocked how you can eventually loosen up to a point where you can make poses you thought were impossible.

6. Makes you sleep better

One of the kinds of advantages after yoga is his ability to make the sleep easier.

Yoga does two things which help you sleep better and deeper. One, it takes you through physically demanding postures to practice Ashtanga and Bikram yoga which is a good example. This exhausts your body and puts your body in a position to re-energize when it is in desperate need of sleep. Second, yoga gives you mental stimulation that induces downtime in your nervous system. This removes tension and repetitive thoughts that keep you awake at night, which means you'll be sleeping better.

7. Strengthen the muscles

You may not know this, but not only do the muscles make us look healthy, but they also protect us from conditions like back pain and arthritis.

One of the easiest ways to create muscle is by practising yoga. The reason it is best is that you are supported by both muscle recovery and bodyweight exercise. Usually, you take yourself to places while you practice yoga where you need to strengthen your muscles.

YOGA SUTRA AND ITS SANSKRIT TERMS

There are over fifty separate English translations of Yoga Sutras, which act as a human monument to how a rich diversity honours Universal Truth. The following translation and commentary is the product of personal familiarity and direct experience with both an authentic yogic tradition and Western culture, psychology and language, refined, tested in fire and integrated over thirty-five years of intense practise (sadhana), rather than the traditional and shallow mode of understanding (emanating from the knowledge of books). This work is dedicated to unveiling the universal message of genuine yoga first published around 2000 years ago by the sage, Patanjali.

Patanjali is not the founder of yoga but the yoga scribe most popularly known. It has become known as the "Yoga Sutras" (sutra means thread) or nearly as popular as the "Yoga Darshana" (yoga vision), which is, in fact, a compendium of an ancient pre-existing oral yoga tradition of practical advice and theoretical significance. The Yoga Sutras' most accepted format consists of four chapters (called padas) written in the Sanskrit language around 2000 years ago in northern India using the terminology of the time, i.e., Samkhya's metaphysical trappings.

The dates assigned to the Sutras Yoga range greatly from 250 BC to 300 AD. 250 AD is quite doubtful, based on a comparative study of the period's associated texts, syntax and simultaneous philosophical ideas. This latter date is a speculation based on the absence before that date of any prior commentary on the Yoga Sutras. What you may say is the Patanjali era was proto-tantric, Buddhist, Jain, Hindu, and eclectic. Since authentic yoga has been mainly an oral tradition (as opposed to a written tradition), the practices precede the texts, but due to the lack of prior literature, it is difficult to know how far ahead.

Most people now believe that yoga rituals, faith, or even the Supreme Spirit (God) upheld by man's beliefs and scriptures, but we will deconstruct it as nonsense. By the life story of the Buddha (who was a yoga practitioner around 500 BCE) and by other accounts these yoga practices may have pre-existed before 1000 BC. Nonetheless, a thorough historical analysis based on style, vocabulary, and literary techniques may reasonably accurately date Patanjali's Yoga Sutras, but such a review goes beyond the scope of this presentation. For our reason, we must accept the entire standard four chapters of the "Yoga Sutras" as authentic (though we acknowledge the dispute as to the possibility of post-humorously adding additional sutras).

While classical Indian historians pay little attention to the linear dimensions of time, it is enough to infer that somewhere around the time of Jesus, plus or minus 200 years ago, the Yoga Sutras were most probably written. We may infer that Patanjali was an educated man who, in his middle or later life, received oral instruction in raj yoga practices and took up yoga practices in remote caves, forests, or river banks which were the most common practice grounds of the time. The yogi Patanjali there obtained the Siddha (perfection) of nirbija samadhi (seedless samadhi), the crown achievement of yoga. As the remote havens of the yogis receded and the true aspirants dwindled, it is believed that Patanjali decided to log the Yoga's most significant teachings which were his guidance and inspiration for enlightenment.

Patanjali's yoga type, as a practice, is non-theistic, not even having the slightest suggestion of worshipping gods, deities, gurus, or holy books; but at the same time, it does not contain any doctrine of atheism. Although this reality has been challenged by self-interested groups, a detailed, objective study of the Yoga Sutras, in particular the discussion of what Patanjali means by the word, "Isvara," will prove to be unquestionable.

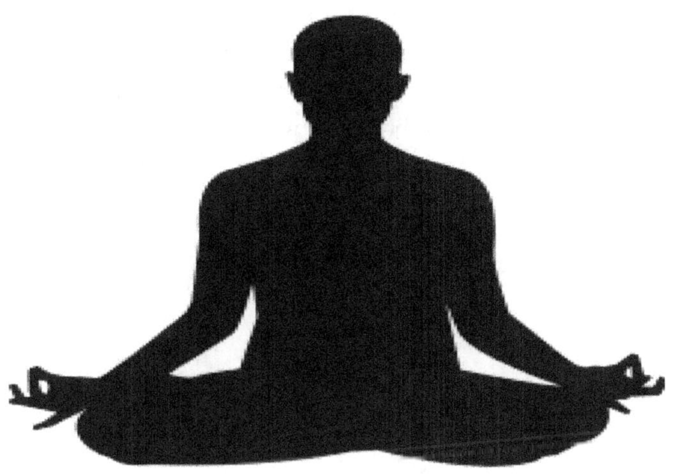

SAMADHI PADA

CONCENTRATION: ITS SPIRITUAL USES

1.*atha yoganushasanam*

Now it's clarified concentration.

2. Yoga restrains the mind (Chitta) from taking different forms (Vrttis)

We need a lot of clarification in this area. What is Chitta and what are those Vrttis, we need to understand. I keep an eye on that. Not having the eyes. Take away the core of the brain in the head, the eyes are still there, the retinœ complete and still the vision, and yet the eyes can not see. So the eyes are just a secondary instrument, not the organ of vision. The centre of viewing is situated in the nerve centre of the brain. Two eyes alone won't be enough. Often a man has his eyes opened to sleep. There is light, and there is the picture, but it needs a third thing; the mind has to be joined to the heart. The eye is the outer tool, so it's the brain centre that we need so mind department. Carriages roll down a street and are not seeing you. Why? Why? Why? Why? If the mind hasn't connected to the hearing organ itself.

First, there's the voice, then the organ, and third, the mind's relation to those two. The mind takes the meaning further in and reveals this to Buddhi, the addressing determinative faculty. The notion of selfishness flashes alongside the reaction. And the combination of action and reaction is introduced to the Purusa, the real Spirit, who perceives an object in this combination. The organs (Indriyas) along with the mind (Manas), the determinative faculty (Buddhi), and egoism (Ahamkara) form the group called the Antahkarana (the inner instrument). They are simply different structures within the mind-stuff, called Chitta. The waves of awareness are called Vrtti in the Chitta.

SADHANA PADA

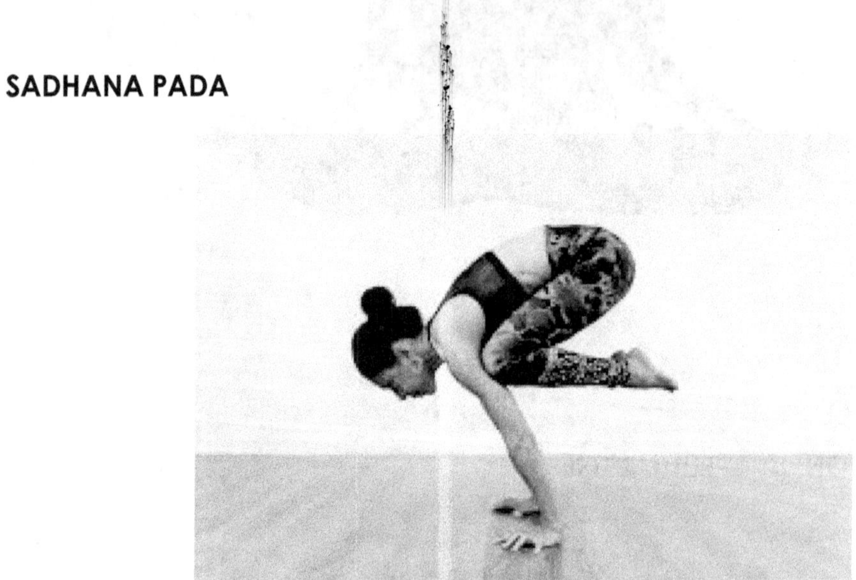

CONCENTRATION - ITS PRACTICE

Mortification, study, and the labour fruits which surrender to God are called Kriya Yoga. The Samadhis we finished our last chapter with are very difficult to attain;

so we have to progressively take them up. The first step is known as Kriya Yoga, the preliminary step. That is to work for Yoga. The organs are the riders, the mind is the reins, the charioteer, the spirit I am the intellect. If a man is naive, he takes up the first part of it, the argumentative war, and reasoning, pro and con.; and when he ends up taking up the Siddhanta, the definitive, concluding. Arriving at the conclusion is not something possible. It needs to be stepped up. Books are infinite in number, and time is short; therefore, this is the essence of wisdom, to take what is required.

VIBHOOTI PADA

THE CHAPTER OF POWERS

We have now come to the chapter which is called the Chapter of Powers.

1. deshabandhashchittasya Dharana

In her view, Dharana sticks to some particular thing. Dharana (concentration) is when the mind holds on to an object, either in the body or outside of the body, and keeps in that state itself.

2. tatra pratyayaikatanata dhyanam

Dhyana is an unbroken knowledge flow toward that individual. The mind tries to think of one thing, to hold on to one particular position, as the top of the head, the heart, etc., and if the mind succeeds in feeling the sensations only through that part of the body, and through no other section, it will be Dharana, and if the mind succeeds in maintaining itself in that state for a while it is called Dhyana (meditation).

3. tad evarthamatranirbhasan svaroopashoonyam iva samadhih

If that, surrendering all forms, only reflects the heart, it is Samadhi. This is when all ways of meditation are giving up. Suppose I was meditating on a book, and slowly managed to concentrate the mind on it, feeling only the inner sensations, meaning Dhyana's condition is called samadhi in any form.

4.trayam ekatra sanyamah

(These) Samyama is three in favour of one piece (when practised). If a man can direct and fix his mind to some particular object, and then hold it there for a long time, separating the object from the inner section, that's Samyama; or Dharana, Dhyana, and Samadhi, one after another, and making one. The form of the thing has gone missing, and only its meaning remains in the brain.

KAIVALYA PADA

INDEPENDENCE

janmaushadhimantratapahsamadhijah siddhayah

By creation, chemical processes, word regulation, mortification, or concentration, the Siddhis (powers) are attained. A man is also born with the Siddhis, powers, of course, from the exercise of the powers he had in his earlier birth. In that birth he is born, as it were, to enjoy their fruits. Kapila, the great father of the Sankhya philosophy, is said to have been a born Siddha, meaning, literally, a good man. The yogis believe they can gain those powers through chemical means. You all know that chemistry originally began as alchemy; men went in search of the philosopher's stone, and the elixirs of life, etc.

At Inidia there had been a sect called the Rasayanas. Their theory was that ideality, intellect, spirituality and faith were all very well, but that the body was the only tool to achieve all of these. When the body breaks out now and then it will take too much more time to reach the mark.

A guy wants to practice Yoga, for example, or he wants to become spiritual. He dies before too much happening. So he takes another body and begins again, then dies, and so on, thus wasting a lot of time on dying and being born again. If the body could be made strong and healthy, we will have so much more time to become spiritual, to get rid of birth and death.

So these Rasayanas suggest, first make the body very solid, and they assume that this body can be made immortal. The hypothesis is that if the mind produces the body, and if it is true that each mind is only one source of that infinite energy, and there is no limit on each outlet receiving any amount of power from outside, why is it difficult for us to keep our bodies all the time? All the bodies we'll ever have will have to be invented. Once that body dies, we will have to create another. If we can do this, can't we just do it without getting out? The statement is entirely right. If we can live and make other bodies after death, why is it impossible for us to have the power to make bodies here without dissolving this body entirely, literally changing it constantly? They also thought that mercury and sulfur provided the most wonderful power and that a man would be able to keep the body as long as he liked by certain of these preparations. Some thought it might bring power to certain substances, such as flying through the air etc.

We owe many of the most excellent therapies of today to the Rasayamas, in particular the use of metals in medicine. Many sects of yogis say many of their leading teachers still exist in their old bodies. Patanjali, the great expert on Yoga, doesn't dispute that.

Potence of words. There are certain sacred words called Mantrams which, when repeated under proper conditions, have the power to produce certain extraordinary powers. We live, day and night, in such a sea of miracles that we think nothing of them. The power of man, the power of words, and the power of the mind are no limits.

To mortify. You may note that mortifications and asceticisms were performed in every religion. In these religious beliefs, the Hindus prefer to go to extremes. You will see men standing up with their hands all their lives, before the willow and death of their life. People sleep standing, day and night until their feet swell, and in this posture, if they live, the legs become so stiff that they can't bend them anymore but have to stand their entire lives. I saw a man raise his hands in this way once and I asked him how he felt when he did it first. He said the torture was horrific. It was such a pain that he had to go to a river and place himself in water, and that allayed the misery a little bit. After a month he hadn't lost much. Capable of attaining powers (Siddhis) through these practices.

Concentrate. Focus. Samadhi is the focus, and it is proper to Yoga; it is the main theme of this study, and it is the highest mean. The previous ones are just secondary, and we can't strive to top by them. Samadhi is our way of getting something and everything.

Glossary of Sanskrit Terms

Advaita ("non-duality"):The teaching that there is only one truth (Atman, Brahman), particularly as found in the Upanishads; see also Vedanta.

Ahimsa ("non-harming"): non-violence against oneself or others in thought or practice.

Ananda ("bliss"): the state of divine happiness that is an integral attribute of the ultimate truth.

Anga ('limb'): a particular Yogic path type, such as the eight limbs of

Ashtanga—asana, Dharana, dhyana, niyama, pranayama, pratyahara, samadhi, Yama.

Angustha: Big toe

Asana ("seat"): a physical posture that originally meant the only posture of meditation, but later this aspect of the Yogic Path was largely developed in Hatha Yoga.

Ardha ('half'): often used in explanations of asana; or half-moon pose of "Ardha Chandrasana."

Atman ("self"): the everlasting transcendental Being, or Spirit — our true existence or personality

Avidya ("ignorance"): The root cause of suffering (Duhkha)

Ayurveda ("knowledge of life"): one of India's main medical systems

Baddha: captured; confined; bound

Bakasana: pose with the crow

Balasana: a pose for children

Bhakti: ("devotion"): Divine or Guru love as a Divine manifestation

Bhakti Yoga: ("devotional yoga"): a major branch of yoga practice, using emotions to communicate with the absolute truth

Bhujangasana: Attitude to the serpent

Brahmacharya (from Brahma and acharya—"Brahmic behaviour): "self-restraint discipline related to sexual behaviour.

Brahman ("what's been expansive"): the ultimate reality

Chakra ("wheel"): a subtle-body psycho-energetic hub

Chaturanga Dandasana: worker poses with four limits

Cit ("consciousness"): The ultimate reality of the super-conscious

Citta ("consciousness"): ordinary consciousness, mind, as opposed to quotation

Danda: ("personnel")

Dandasana: Posture of the staff

Drishti: ('view/sight'): a gaze point such as at the tip of the nose or between the eyebrows

Gayatri-mantra: a famous Vedic mantra, one of the oldest traditions of yoga

Guna ('quality'): refers to each of the three primary 'qualities' or constituents of nature – tamas (the inertia principle), rajas (the dynamic principle), and sattva (the lucidity principle)

Hasta: right hand

Hatha Yoga ('strong yoga'): a major branch of yoga that highlights the physical aspects of the journey, especially postures (asana) and relaxation techniques (shodhana), but also breath control (Pranayama).

Hatha-Yoga-Pradipika ("Light upon Hatha Yoga"): one of the classical manuals of Hatha Yoga

Janu: Knee Learn

Jivan-mukti ("living liberation"): release state when embodied

Jnana ("wisdom/knowledge"): earthly understanding and world-transcendent wisdom.

Kali: The goddess embodying the Divine's fiery dimension

Kali-yuga: the dark age of deterioration in spirit and morale, believed to be existing now. An age in which Light is desperately needed.

Karma ("action"): any type of operation

Karma Yoga ("Action Yoga"): the transformative road to self-transcendent practice.

Karna: Ore

Kona ("angle"): as in Konasana Baddha (bound angle pose)

Kosha ("casing"): any of the five envelopes that cover the transcendental Self

Kumbhaka ('pot-like'): retention of breath during Pranayama

Kundalini-shakti ("coiled power"): the serpent power or divine energy that resides at the body's lowest energetic core to be awakened and directed to the crown core to fully awaken.

Kundalini Yoga: The yogic route that focuses on kundalini energy as a means of deliverance

Mantra: a sacred sound or word that has a transformative effect, such as om or om Namah Shivaya

Mantra Yoga: the yogic path utilizing mantras as the primary means of practice

Matsyendra ("Lord of Fishes"): an early Tantric master — the seated twist is named after him

Maya ("the one who measures"): The illusory representation of consciousness

Face: Muhka

Nada ("sound"): the inner sound, as can be heard in the Nada Yoga practice by closing the ear flaps

Nadi ("conduit"): one of the 72,000 subtle channels through which the life force (prana) flows, the three most prominent of which are the Ida-Nadi, Pingala-Nadi and sushumnanadi.

Nadi Shodhana (" channel cleansing): "the practice of purifying the conduits, especially through breath control, which moves the body's subtle energies (Pranayama)

Namaskara: greeting or salutation

Nava: boat

Niyama (" self-restraint): "the second limb of Patanjali's Eightfold Path, which consists of purity (saucha), contentment (santosha), austerity (tapas), study (svadhyaya), and dedication to the Lord (Ishvara-pranidhana)

Om: the first mantra that symbolizes the final truth

Pachima: To the west

Pada: socle

Padma: bigots

Patanjali: The Sutras Yoga Compiler

Prana ("life / breath"): the body maintaining life-force

Pranayama (from prana and Ayama): The practice of prana movement by breathing

Pratyahara ("withdrawal"): sensory suppression, 5th limb (anga) of the Eightfold Path of

Patanjali

Parsva: front

Parivrtta: Turned or twisted

Prasarita: wide range

Purusha: the soul or the transcendental self (atman)

Raja: King

Sadhana ("accomplishment"): Spiritual practice leading to siddhi ("perfection" or "accomplishment");

Samadhi ("to bring together"): the state in which the meditator is one with the object of meditation, the eighth limb (anga) of Patanjali's Eightfold Path

Samsara: The world of inconstant transition, as opposed to the true truth

Samskara: the subconscious impression left behind by any act of volition; similar to a predisposition to other actions which lead to Karma

Sat ("being / reality / truth"): absolute realization

Satya ("fact/truthfulness"): fact, the absolute reality designation; also the practice of truthfulness, which is an element of moral discipline (Yama)

Shakti ("power"): the supreme feminine, artistic element of Nature

Shakti-pata ("descent of power"): the cycle of initiation by an experienced or even enlightened adept (Siddha) through the transmission of shakti

Shankara: the adept of the eighth century who was the main practitioner of non-dualism (Advaita Vedanta)

Sirsasana: chief executive

Shiva ('The Benign One'): the Almighty, the Unmanifested Power

Shiva-Sutra ('Shiva's Aphorisms'): like Patanjali's Yoga Sutras, a classical yoga work taught in the Cashmir Shaivism; written by Vasugupta (ninth century C.E.)

Shodhana ("cleansing/purification"): a form of Hatha Yoga purification practice

Shraddha ("faith"): a condition of pure and continuous confidence

Siddha ("accomplished"): an experienced Tantric

Siddha Yoga: A classification attributed to Kashmiri Shaivism yoga in particular, as taught by Swami Muktananda

Spanda ('vibration'): the perception of Kashmir's Shaivism that absolute truth itself 'vibrates;' a non-sequential pulse of development

Supta: to sleep, to lie down;

Surya: Sun Shine

Sushumna-Nadi: the central prana current in or through which the strength of the serpent (kundalini ushakti) will rise to the crown chakra

Sutra ('thread'): a short verse; a collection of aphoristic statements, such as the Yoga Sutras of Patanjali or the Shiva-Sutra of Vasugupta

Svana: ('Dog")

Tantra ("loom" or "to weave"): Sanskrit work containing Tantric teachings; the Tantrism tradition in which the human body is seen as the Supreme's condensation

Tapas ("glow/heat"): restraint, a fire that purifies discipline

Tattva ("thatness"): a fact or reality; a particular category of existence; the way universal consciousness stepped down in vibration to create the physical world — the "Tattvas"

Tri: three

Upanishad ("sitting close"): a kind of scripture that reflects revealed wisdom

Upavistha: Sits

Urdhva: Upstream

Utthita: Spread

Vairagya: ("committal")

Vasistasana: balance of the side-arms

LEARNING ABOUT PHYSICAL, EMOTIONAL, ATTITUDE IN YOGIC LIFESTYLE

We also learned that body disorder is caused by the primary cause (mad thought patterns). If the source of this primary cause is annihilated then it will cure all diseases. How can we get this done? If the mind becomes filled with true Satvagu, then Prāa Vāyu will begin to circulate freely in the body, the food taken will be properly digested and thus there will be no illnesses. The Yoga Vāsistha has described this splendidly. This is also consistent with the Yama and niyama of Patañjali mentioned in the preceding unit under Aāāga Yoga.

Rules and regulations (ācāra and vicāra)

Avoid actions such as:

1. Eating unhealthy food

2. Living in unsanitary places

3. Do things over unreasonable hours

4. Association with the Bad

5. Longing after stuff wrong

6. Wrong wishes and bad thoughts

Development of Sattvaguṇa

In an average man, there is a combination of the three guas (Sattva, Rājas, and Tamas). Tamas and Rājas force a man down; Sattva pushes a man up. Tamas and Rājas contribute to serfdom; Sattva helps to make redemption come about. Discipline yourself, and cultivate the Sattva. When the mind is Sāttvika there is calmness in it. Divine light will only enter when the mind is serene and joyful.

The Sāttvika man regulates the senses, performs selfless service, and performs Japa, prā halfāyāma, concentration, reflection, self-analysis, and "Who am I?" inquiry, there is no desire for sensual objects. He has a burning desire for achievement by mok (salvation). He is modest, gracious, compassionate, tolerant and devout. A small personality of his is lost. The rājasika man is arrogant, intolerant, self-sustaining, lustful, hot-tempered, covetous and jealous. He works both for his glory and prestige, and for self-enlargement. His small personality is changing. The guas and the karmas have an intimate relationship. The essence of karmas is based upon the guas' existence.

A man will do noble deeds at Sāttvika. A Rājasika and Tāmasika man will commit non-virtue acts. It is the quiz gu who guides a man to act. The Brahman or The Self is less about behaviour. He is the observer- the silent witness. Virtuous existence helps the aspirant to achieve the highest state of supra-consciousness (Nirvikalpa Samādhi), in which the seer and the sighted are combined into one; the meditator and the meditated become identical.

The Bhagvadgītā lists the virtues here:

1. Fearlessness (Abhayam)

Among the Divine virtues lies, above all, fearlessness. Fear is an outcome of Ignorance. Identification of the body causes fear. Fear is caused by blind attachment to the body, wife, husband, kids, home, property etc. The sage who discovered that he was himself is fearless. "Whoever knows the Peace of Brahman (God), from which all words and mind become helpless, fears nothing. "—Taittirīya Upaniad Fear can be eliminated by continuous thought of the eternal and all-blissful essence of the Soul. If you live a life of integrity and truthfulness, if you devotedly follow the scriptural precepts, if you lead a life of correct behaviour, and if you always remember God, you become fearless.

2. The purity of heart (Satvasaṁśuddhiḥ)

It includes purity of knowledge, purity of life or purity of heart, purity of mind, i.e. giving up stealing, deceit, untruth, and the like in all dealings with the people, and doing transactions with complete honesty and integrity is the purity of heart. A pure mind can not be achieved without dedication to the Lord.

3. Steadfastness in knowledge and Yoga (Jñāna Yogavyavasthitiḥ)

Understanding the essence of the Self as taught in the scriptures and by the preceptor, self-realization is insight by meditation on the great phrase of Upaniad, "I am Brahman" (Aham Brahmāsmi). Yoga is the union of the human soul with the Supreme Being; it is the realization of the Self by self-restraint or sensory awareness, by concentration and meditation.

4. Almsgiving (Dāna)

Distributing food, clothes, etc. to the degree that, according to one's means, it is within one's ability and expertise, to those who are deprived of it and in need. A man of kindness hastens to console the sick and supports the poor.

5. Control of the senses (Dama)

It requires self-restraint, self-control, and control of the sensory outside. The practice of self-regulation annihilates the bond between the senses and the sources of the senses. He/she keeps the senses under the strictest control and is balanced in one's diet, tests the outgoing habits of the mental and senses. He/she causes senses and mindset to turn back to their source.

For them, even moderation or controlled and balanced life would be self-restraint, as householders can not exercise complete regulation of the senses. The practice of self-control involves compassion, harmlessness, honesty, steadfastness and patience.

6. Study of scriptures (Svādhyāya)

Research the Vedas or any other scripture you believe in to attain the 'unseen fruits,' such as the Quran, the Scriptures, etc. It also involves the self-analysis and self-reflection attempts to know yourself.

7. Austerity (Tapas)

True tapas is a meditation on the Self. It fixes the mind either upon the Ultimate Truth or on the Self. It is about shifting one 's attention to the soul. Respect for the gods, the twice-born, the teachers, and the wise, observance of modesty, innocence, celibacy, and non-injury are called body austerities (tapas, or self-discipline).

A discourse that does not cause excitement, factual, friendly and useful, the practice of learning the Vedas, is called speech austerity. One should be talking true; one should be talking pleasingly. One does not speak the real but not the good nor the nice but the fake.

8. Straightforwardness (Ārjavam)

That's conducive to awareness attainment. The aspirant should always be straight, upright or open. One 's mindset should be straightforwardness. Only a man who is honest and real can be straightforward. People admire a man like that who is respected by everyone. He finds success in all his endeavours. He never hides the truth or reality.

9. Non-violence (Ahiṁsā)

No harm to any person-man or animal in mind, speech, and deed. The powers of the Rājas are suppressed by refraining from harming living beings. Ahi affairs are categorized as emotional, physical, and verbal.

10. Truth (Satyam)

To talk of things as they are without offensive words or lies being spoken. These include self-restraint, lack of envy, pardon, tolerance, resilience and kindness.

11. Absence of anger (Akrodha)

There is no outrage when he is insulted, rebuked or battered, that is, except under the extreme provocation.

12. Renunciation (Tyāgaḥ)

To give up; to give up the vāsanās egotism and the fruits of action. Charity is also tyâga.

13. Peacefulness (Śānti): Serenity of the mind or tranquillity

14. Absence of crookedness/backbiting (Apaisunam)

Aversion to slander, and lack of narrowness of mind.

15. Compassion towards beings (Dayā)

Compassion for troubled people. A Merciful Man has a tender heart. He lives only for the love of the world. Compassion implies the recognition of harmony or oneness with other beings.

16. Freedom from covetousness (Aloluptvam)

Non-friendliness. The senses are not disturbed or agitated when they come into contact with their respective objects; rather, they are removed from the objects of the senses just as the tortoise limbs are removed by it into their shell.

17. Gentleness/tenderness (Mārdavam)

18. Modesty (Hrih)- It is shameful to conduct acts contrary to the laws of the Vedas or other texts.

19. Absence of fickleness (Acāpalam)

Not thinking pointlessly. Not changing your hands and legs in vain. Stop futile behaviour.

20. Vigour (Tejas)

Vigour, strength, splendour. The aspirant bent upon salvation attainment marches confidently on the spiritual path. Nothing can threaten him, or slacken his development. This unbraked development towards the knowledge of the Self or the Absolute is lustre. She surmounts downward pull from Tamas.

21. Forgiveness (Kṣamā)

And when he is insulted, rebuked, or beaten, he who is born with this virtue does not show indignation while he is powerful enough to take revenge. The insult or wound, or even happiness or sorrow, does not affect him.

22. Fortitude (Dhṛti)

In himself, the sage absorbs all the calamities. He is steadfast even though he finds himself in very challenging and most adverse circumstances. This is a particular sāttvika or state of mind that eliminates stress or fatigue from the body and senses as they fall. An aspirant born with this divine quality never becomes disheartened, even though under extreme trials and tribulations and hardships. Dhivelti is a divine tonic in a state of low or dejected spirits when the body and the senses.

23. Cleanliness/purity (Saucam)

There are two forms of this: external, and internal. External cleanliness is obtained by soil and water, soap and so on. It involves the cleanliness of the environment, the body, the clothes etc. Internal Purity: Intellect and mind are free from Maya; free from deceit, desire, rage, envy, vanity, resentment, hypocrisy, likes, and dislikes. Purity is attained by the practice of celibacy, pardon, goodness, charity, modesty, integrity, devotion, self-indulgence, compassion, etc.

24. Absence of hatred/enmity (Adroha)

Free the malice. It includes a lack of desire to wound others.

25. Absence of overweening pride (Atimānitā)

Atimânitā is exceptionally proud. A proud man believes he is superior to others and deserving of being respected by others.

YOGIC NUTRITIONAL DIET AND ITS DISCUSSION ON HEALTHY LIVING

Āhāra or Yogic diet

Dieting is catching up among the rich, even in India-for better looks, of course; much less for health. It shuns processed foods high in calories. There is also a battle between the palate and the need for a slimming down. The Yogic conception of food takes into account the total dimension of human life. We all possess prā lie, mind, intellect, emotions, and the spiritual dimension of freedom besides the atoms and molecules from which our gross physical body is created.

Yoga is the mechanism by which we introduce an integration of the entire personality at all of these stages. If the endurance of the body is to be established, the prāa should be brought into a nice balance, the mind should be relaxed, the energy balanced and the intellect regulated. Thus, a 'healthy diet' according to Yoga is the diet the maintains equilibrium at all stages. Only those diets may assist in the creation of a holistic way of life and personality. Let's see how the ancient sages came to the idea of a good diet and define their general characteristics.

Food Classification

Yoga classifies food in the primarily Tāmasika, Rājasika, and Sātvika foods into three groups (similar to human classification).

Rājasika Foods

Rājasika likes ka Riu (bitter), amla (sour), lava ripe (saline), ati u ripe (hot steam), tīka (burning). It is called Rājasika what stimulates the nervous system, accelerates metabolism and activates that. Examples of this include coffee, tea, tobacco. Green chillies and pepper are considered Rājasika but the dried red chillies seem to be more Tāmasika.

The Rájasika are luxury wines. These Rājasika foods can energize but not offer strong balanced energy. They tend to stimulate and drive the organism to increase its pace and to engage more in physical activity, sensual pleasures, and comfort. Spiced and cooked to perfection with plenty of rich sauces, it tempts one to eat more and draws attention to the savour of the food and away from the internal signals. It is known that a moving, violent worldly form of operation fits the rulers, the armed powers, and those concerned with political issues — who deal with dominance, power, and war.

In fact, in some of the Indian traditions, the castes that performed such roles – the Rajputs (literally "son of the King") were specifically permitted to take meat and wine, while the Brāhmaa, who is not a ruler but a scholar, teacher, and spiritual seeker, has always been forbidden to take these Rājasika foods. Such a diet, no doubt, produces brilliant energies within a person and keeps all vigorous men restlessly trying to satisfy their uncontrolled passions and desires; thus they lead the eater in their final reactions to a productive life of 'pain, sorrow, and disease.'

Sātvika Foods

Satva (purity), Bala (stamina strength), rogya (health), Sukha (happiness), and Prīti (happiness and good appetite) are called Sāttvika foods that enhance the āyu al (life and vitality). These foods are like Rasyā (savoury), like Snigdhā (oleaginous), like Sthirā (substantial), like Hadjā (pleasant), and like Sāttvika. Unlike Tāmasika and Rājasika foods, foods that are fresh, organic, edible, of good quality, but mild in spices, never overcooked or undercooked, are experienced as giving calm alertness and at the same time a quiet state of energy. Such food is known as Sātvika.

They're supposed to nourish consciousness. They not only provide nourishment for the body but they do not adversely affect the overall energy level. They add vitality to the total system by bringing a fine, harmonious equilibrium of energy states into the food itself. They don't pull or weigh energy out of the body; they don't make it heavy; they don't irritate or push it beyond their capacity. Instead, they have a precise nutritional balance and do not produce excessive waste. Such foods are the most likely to be considered a Sātvika. They are the ones that are likely to bring lightness, alertness, energy and clear consciousness to the body. The Sāttvika food gives power from inside.

In comparison, Rājasika foods offer power to the muscles and give the impression that one's energy comes from the meal, one has consumed. Food Sāttvika is fresh fruit, wholesome grains, and fresh milk from a cow. It is considered ideal raw milk only harvested from a good cow. If it is held long until it is eaten, however, then it must be heated to its boiling point. Buffalo milk is considered more Rājasika because it is heavier and more fattening. Of course, whatever milk becomes sour or spoiled tends to acquire Tāmasika land.

When describing the natural taste of particular types of food that are accepted and liked by good men of spiritual urges (Sattva), it is said that they only like those diets that increase vitality (including yuu) and not pure bulk; that supplies the energy for meditative purposes (Vīrya); that increases and unfolds the secret power (Bala) to resist sensory object temptations; that provides goo, Such creative people, in short, just enjoy their love for pure and wholesome food.

Āhāra vihāra – the key is moderation

He who is healthy in his cooking, eating, working and leisure activities by practising Yoga will relieve all material pains. Yukta-āhāra-vihārasya, one whose food and enjoyment are regulated – āhāra (lit. food) means all that is taken in, āhāra, which also means food, involves mental 'food as well as the connections we build in our sense organs and the people we are associated with. Vihāra means pleasures and also yukta-that one whose dedication (ceā) is gentle, does not work excessively; karmasu in works (not workaholics); likewise yukta-svapna-avabodhasya, of one whose normal sleep (svapna) and wakefulness (avabodha) will solve all worldly pains and sorrows.

ANCIENT PRINCIPLE ON MUDRAS AND ITS SCIENTIFIC KNOWLEDGE

In Sanskrit, the word mudra is translated as 'gesture' or 'attitude.' Mudras can be defined as mental, emotional, devotional, and aesthetic gestures or attitudes.Yogis have experienced mudras as attitudes of energy flow intended to connect individual pranic force with universal or cosmic force." Kularnava Tantra traces the word mudra to the root mud which means 'delight' or 'pleasure' and gravity, the causal type of dru which means 'to draw out.' Mudra is also known as 'seal,' 'short-cut' or 'circuit bypass.'

GYANA AND CHIN MUDRAS

Gyana Mudra (psychic gesture of knowledge)

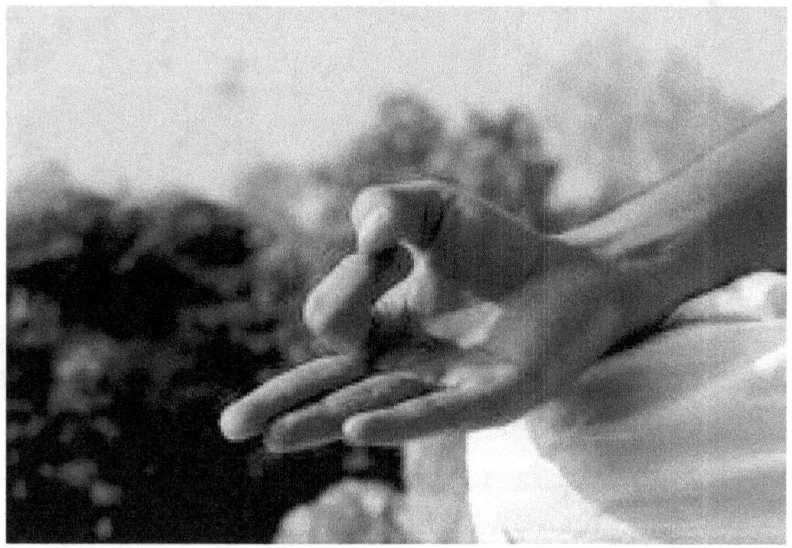

Assume a relaxing meditation pose. Fold the index fingers so that they meet the thumbs' inner base. Straighten each hand's other three fingers so that they are relaxed and slightly apart. Put the hands on the knees with the palms facing downwards.

Chin Mudra (psychic gesture of consciousness)

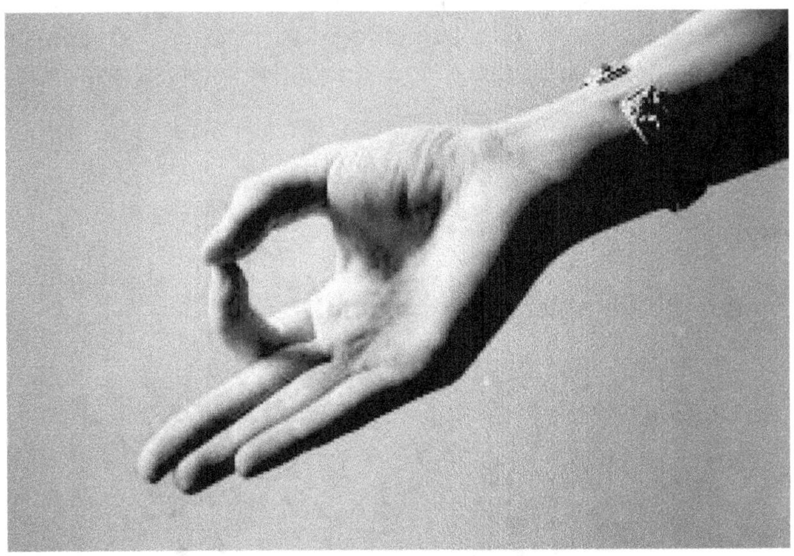

Chin mudra is performed in the same way as gyana mudra except that both hands 'palms face upwards, with the hands' back resting on the feet.

Sequence: One of those two mudras should be followed while practising meditation unless otherwise stated.

Benefits: gyana mudra and chin mudra are simple yet essential psycho neural finger locks that make meditation asanas more effective. Hand palms and fingers have various nerve root endings that continuously emit energy. When the finger touches the thumb a circuit is generated that allows the energy that would normally dissipate into the atmosphere to move back to the body and up to the thumb.

This Nadi is known as the secret nadi or Gupta. Sensitizing this channel helps to activate the mooladhara chakra energies. In chin mudra, when the palms face upwards, the chest region is opened. The practitioner may perceive this as a sense of lightness and receptivity that is absent in the practice of gyana mudra.

Variation: Gyana and chin mudras are often done by touching and forming a circle with thumb tip and index finger. Beginners can find this variation less secure for extended periods of meditation because the thumb and index finger appear to separate more easily when body consciousness is lost. Otherwise, this variation would be as successful as the fundamental position.

Practice note: The effect of chin or gyana mudras is very subtle and it takes great sensitivity on the part of the practitioner to perceive the defined shift in consciousness. However, with practice, the mind becomes accustomed to the mudra, and when it is embraced, the signal to enter a meditative state is transmitted.

BHAIRAVA MUDRA

Bhairava Mudra (fierce or terrifying attitude)

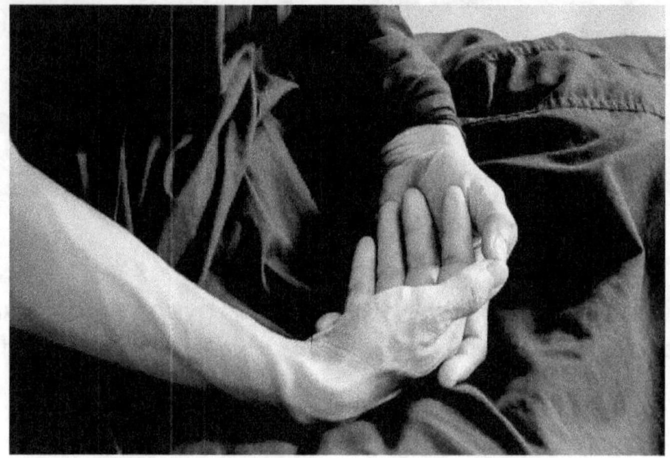

Assume a relaxed sitting pose, with straight head and neck. Position the right hand over the left hand so that the palms of both hands face up. Then both hands recline in the lap. Close the eyes and relax, leaving the whole body motionless.

Variation: The procedure is called Bhairavi mudra when the left hand is put over the right. Bhairavi is the female equivalent to Bhairava.

Note: Bhairava is the fearsome or frightening form of Lord Shiva, the aspect that is responsible for the destruction of the world. Both hands represent ida and Pingala nadis, and the union of the soul with the supreme consciousness. Bhairava mudra is used in prana mudra, and can also be used in pranayama and meditation.

PRANA MUDRA

Prana Mudra (invocation of energy)

Sit in any relaxed meditation pose, preferably in bhairava mudra padmasana or Siddha / Siddha yoni asana. Close your eyes and relax your entire body, especially your abdomen, your arms and your hands.

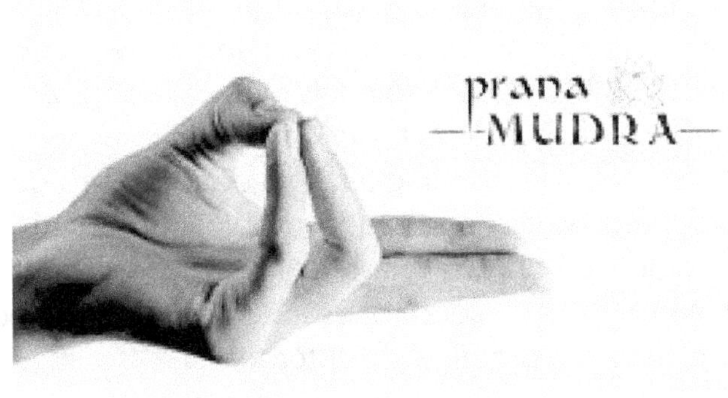

Step I: keeping the eyes closed, inhaling and exhaling as intensely as possible, contracting the abdominal muscles to expel as much air as possible from the lungs. Perform moola bandha with the breath held outside while focussing on perineum mooladhara chakra. Hold out the air as long as it is convenient.

Step 2: Unleash moola bandha. Inhale slowly and deeply, stretching the belly to draw as much oxygen into the lungs as possible. Simultaneously raise your hands so they are in front of the navel. The hands should be open with the fingers pointing towards each other but not touching one another, and the palms facing the trunk of the body. Hand motion should be combined with abdominal inhalation. His arms and hands should relax. Try to feel the prana or essential energy in the spinal column flowing from the mooladhara chakra to the Manipura chakra as you inhale it from the abdomen.

Step 3: Begin inhalation by widening the chest and elevating the hands right up to the heart centre. Try to feel the pranic energy pulled from Manipura into Anahata chakra when you are inhaling.

Step 4: Draw even more air into the lungs by gently elevating the shoulders, and feel the prana drawn to vishuddhi. Raise hands to the front of the mouth, in sync with the wind.

Step 5: Hold the air inside while you extend your arms toward your side. The hands in the final position must be level with the feet, the arms extended out but not straight and the palms turned upward. Felt that prana spread like a wave to Ajna, Bindu, and sahasrara chakras. Focus on the sahasrara chakra and try to imagine an aura of pure light from the head. Thought that the whole being radiates the vibrations of harmony to all things. Maintain this place as long as possible, without any lung pressure. Repeat steps 4, 3, 2, 1, and return slowly while exhaling to start place. Feel the prana steadily descending through each chakra during exhalation, until it reaches mooladhara. At the end of the exhalation perform moola bandha and focus on the mooladhara chakra. The entire body then naturally relaxes and breathes. Visualize the breath as a stream of ascending and descending white light within Sushumna Nadi once the practice is mastered.

Breathing: Slowly increase inhalation, retention, and time to exhale. Look out not to strain the lungs.

Consciousness: The consciousness should pass in a smooth and continuous flow from mooladhara to Sahasrara and back 452 to mooladhara, in sync with the breath and the elevation and lowering of hands.

Sequence: prana mudra is best done after asana and pranayama and before meditation but it can also be performed at any time.

Time of practice: The prana mudra is preferably done at sunrise when facing the sun.

Benefits: Prana mudra awakens and distributes, throughout the body, the latent prana shakti, essential energy, and increases power, health and trust. It creates knowledge of the pranic system, the nadis and chakras, and the gradual flow of prana through the body. It instils an inner attitude of harmony and equanimity by adopting an outward attitude of offering and receiving energy from and to the celestial source. Prana mudra is also known to be a pranayama ritual that elevates prana by facilitating proper respiration.

Practice Note: Remember to return prana to mooladhara at the end of the session.

Note: This practice is also known as Shanti mudra and is the mudra of goodwill.

A scientific look at mudras

Scientifically speaking, mudras offer a way of accessing and manipulating the unconscious reflexes and innate, instinctive behaviour patterns that arise across the brain stem in the primitive brain regions. The link in a subtle, non-intellectual way to those places. -- mudra creates another relation and has a correspondingly different impact on body, mind and prana. The goal is to create fixed, repeated postures and movements that can snap the practitioner out of instinctive behaviour patterns and establish a more sophisticated awareness.

DIFFERENT TYPES OF PRANAYAMA

Pranayama is a combination of two Sanskrit words: prana means "vitality,""essence" or "strength of life" and Ayama means "mastery,""order" or "regulation." Thus pranayama is the mastery of life force. Pranayama is also the control of breath delays or the transition from exhalation to inhalation to exhalation. A variety of ways to use breath are available: relaxing the nervous system, strengthening the healthy body, and helping with meditation.

Pranayama, which means power or interaction with the prana (Life Force), induces quietness within the body. Reflections become simpler and more concentrated, without the slightest ripple, like a stream. Pranayama isn't just "breath management," we have some voluntary control over his breath one thing. Initially, though, we don't have access to regulate other bodily functions, such as the operation of organs like the heart. These roles are autonomous. By subtle manipulation of the breath, by watching its rhythm, by paying attention to the spaces between the breathes, we can begin to note the movement of prana, the Life Force itself. This is the proper purpose of Pranayama-not to raise lung capacity or hold the breath for long periods.

Nadi Suddhi

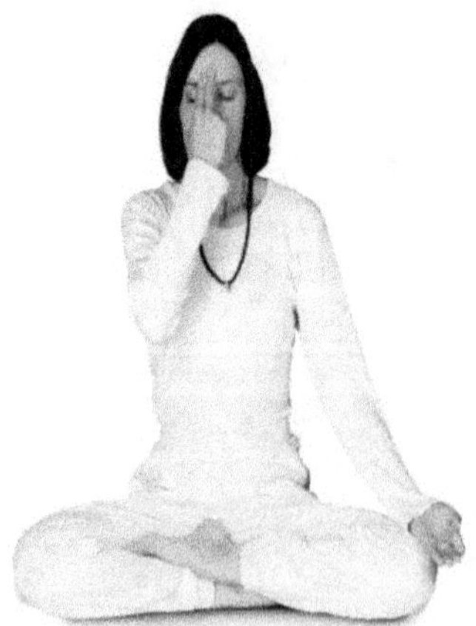

But you should clean the Nadis before you start practising pranayama. Only then can you obtain the full value from the Pranayama. Cleansing the Nadi (Nadi-Suddhi) is either Samanu or Nirmanu — that is, with or without the use of Bija.

The Yogi in Padmasana or Siddhasana, according to the first form, offers his prayers to the Guru and meditates upon it. Via Bija's Ida, Kumbhaka 64 times with Bija's Japa, and then 32 times via Bija's solar Nadi and Japa, he meditates on 'Yang' (y: ú) 16 times.

Fire emerges from Manipura and unites with Prithvi. Then follows the inhalation of the solar Nadi 16 times with the Vahni Bija 'Rang' (rú), Kumbhaka 64 times with the Bija Japa, followed by an exhalation of the Bija 32 times with the lunar Nadi and Japa. Then he meditates on the celestial light, looking at the tip of the nose, and Ida inhales the Bija 'Thang' (Yú) with Japa 16 times. Kumbhaka is performed 64 times using the Vang Bija (v: ú). He feels he's nectar-flooded and assumes the Nadis have been washed off. He exhales Pingala's Bija 'Lang' (l: ú) with Japa 32 times, and thus finds himself improved. Now I'll just tell you some important exercises that are useful in awakening the Kundalini.

1. Sukha Purvaka

(Easy Comfortable Pranayama)

If sitting in Siddhasana or Padmasana. Place your thumb straight into the nostril. Inhale through the left nostril (Puraka), until you slowly count 3 Oms. Imagine drawing the Prana in the atmosphere along with the breeze. In practice, you'll feel like you're drawing Prana. Then close your left nostril with both small and ring fingers on your right hand. Keep the breath running until you count to 12 Oms. Send the current down into the Muladhara Chakra. Feel the nerve-current hitting at the awakening of the Muladhara Chakra and Kundalini. Remove the right thumb, then exhale through the right nostril until you count 6 Oms. Inhale, catch, and exhale through the right nostril, again.

All the six processes listed above form one Pranayama. First, do 6 Pranayamas in the morning and 6 in the evening. Gradually increase it to 20 Pranayamas for each sitting. The ratio between inhalation, hold and exhalation is 1:4:2. You should be gradually rising the Kumbhaka Time. Be patient when you can do the Kumbhaka comfortably. Hurry not to be in. Please note to be polite. Contract butt and Mula Bandha do too. Focus on the Chakra, and do meditation on Kundalini. That is the bulk of the workout. Deep concentration plays an important part in awakening Kundalini in this Pranayama. If the degree of focus is high, and Kundalini is easily awakened when practised daily. This exercise eliminates all pathogens, purifies the Nadis, stabilizes the wandering mind, enhances digestion and circulation, aids Brahmacharya and awakens Kundalini. Any impurities in the body are thrown out.

2. Bhastrika

The fast sequence of forcible expulsions is a feature of this exercise. 'Bhastrika' in Sanskrit means the 'bellows.' Just like a blacksmith blows his bellows rapidly, so you can inhale and exhale quickly too. Sit your number one at Asana. Place your mouth tight. Inhale and exhale 20 times more rapidly than the bellows do. The chest dilates and expands constantly, as you inhale and exhale. When you practice the Pranayama a hissing sound is produced.

You should start with a swift succession of forcible breath expulsions after each other. After 20 such expulsions, take a deep inhalation and hold the air as long as you can safely do it, then exhale slowly. One round of Bhastrika. Start for a round with 10 expulsions, and eventually raise it to about 20 or 25. Even the Kumbhaka period should be gradual, and careful. Rest after one round, and start again and again in the next round.

Do 3 rounds in the beginning and after the correct practice does 20 rounds in the morning and 20 rounds in the evening. This Pranayama is performed after partial closure of the glottis by advanced students. They don't make a potent noise like the beginners. In a standing stance, they can do it too. Bhastrika prevents inflammation of the lungs, raises gastric fire, kills phlegm and all diseases of the nose and lung, eradicates asthma, ingestion and other illnesses caused by excessive wind, bile and phlegm. She gives warmth to the body. It is the most powerful of all the Pranayama exercises that take place. It helps Prana to burst through the Three Granthis. Many other benefits of Sukha Purvaka Pranayama also are obtained in this exercise.

3. Suryabheda

Sit on Padmasana or Siddhasana. Cover their doors. Hold your right ring and fingertips attached to your left nostril. Slowly inhale without making any sound, so long as you can do it comfortably through the right nostril. Then close your right thumb to the nostril and hold back the breath by pressing the chin tightly to the chest (Jalandhara Bandha). Keep the breath, until unexpectedly the hair roots (hair follicles) ooze. At the very beginning, the point is not attainable. You will need to step up the Kumbhaka cycle gradually. That is the limit of the sphere of practice in Suryabheda Kumbhaka. Unblock Bandha in Jalandhara. Then exhale very slowly, closing the right nostril with the thumb, without making any sound through the left nostril.

4.Ujjayi

Sit back in your usual Asana. Place your mouth tight. Inhale slowly from both nostrils, a smooth, standardized way. Hold the air as long as you can, then exhale slowly through the left nostril by closing the right nostril with the right thumb. When you inhale, your chest expands. Due to the partial closing of the glottis a peculiar sound is produced during inhalation. The sound should be of a moderate and consistent pitch when inhaling. And it should be constant as well.

This Kumbhaka can also be done walking or standing. You should slowly exhale from both nostrils, rather than exhale through the left nostril. This takes place in the head of the sun. The practitioner gets cute. The gastric fire is gaining ground. It is doing away with the neck's phlegm. It treats pulmonary disorders of all sorts, asthma, consumption and. All ailments caused by inhalation of insufficient oxygen and heart failure are healed. All the works are performed by Ujjayi Pranayama. No phlegm infections, nerves, spleen enlargement, dyspepsia, dysentery, vomiting, cough, or fever strike the practitioner. Carry out Ujjayi to annihilate decline and death.

SURYANAMASKAR AND ITS BENEFITS

The Surya Namaskar, better known as Surya Namskar or Sun or Sun Salutation Prostrations, is one of the best exercises people can do. The benefits provided by such activities are unique and exceptional. This is a tradition based on yoga, and it's customary to perform Surya Namaskar after performing loosening yoga exercises. The human being can be thought to consist of 'Pancha kosas' (or five sheaths), consisting of sheaths Annamaya (or Body), Pranamaya (or Breath), Manomaya (or Mind), Vijnanamaya (or Intellect) and Anandamaya (or Bliss). These same five kosas can be further divided into Gross (or Sthula), Annamaya or body sheath, Subtle (or Sukshma) composed of pranic, mental, and intellectual sheaths, and Causal (or Karana), the Bliss sheath.

Properly done Surya Namaskar impacts and affects all five sheaths – the body, air, mind, intellect, and bliss – thus giving benefits to the performers of those exercises for the Sthula (Gross), Sukshma (subtle), and Kaarina (Causal) bodies. Although traditional exercises of all types including aerobic, weight lifting, walking, jogging and running are designed to bring benefits to the physical body and its various component organs including joints and muscles, Surya Namaskar offers holistic benefits by working on the entire hu's physical body, prana (breathing), mind, intellect, and bliss components (or kosas) In that sense, Surya Namaskar can be regarded as a tool for personality development and must be included in one's wellness program

Namaskar:

Usually, the Surya Namaskar is performed early in the morning, facing Sun rising in the sky. The Namskar is done in 12 steps, each with its pose (including posture and shape) with its breathing pattern (inhalation or exhalation) and mantra.

The Surya Namaskar Postures and Breathing Patterns:

The 12 postures are:

1. Stand facing the Sun with palms crossed, and both thumbs touching the heart.

Inhale as the hands rise and exhale as the hands slip to the bottom of the chest.

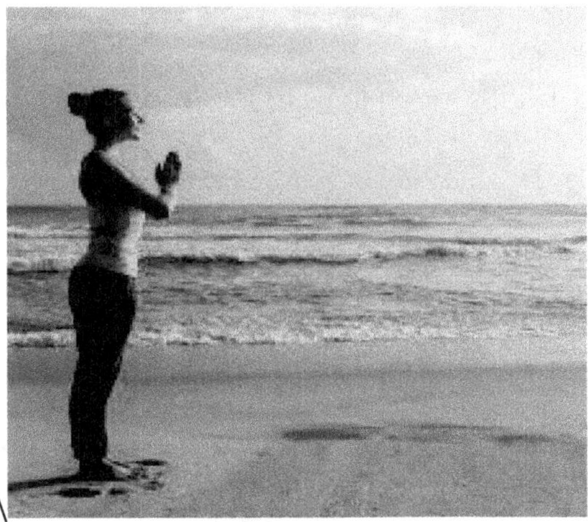

2. Heave up your palms, feet firmly on the deck, lean backwards, stretch your arms wide.

Breathing: Breathing in

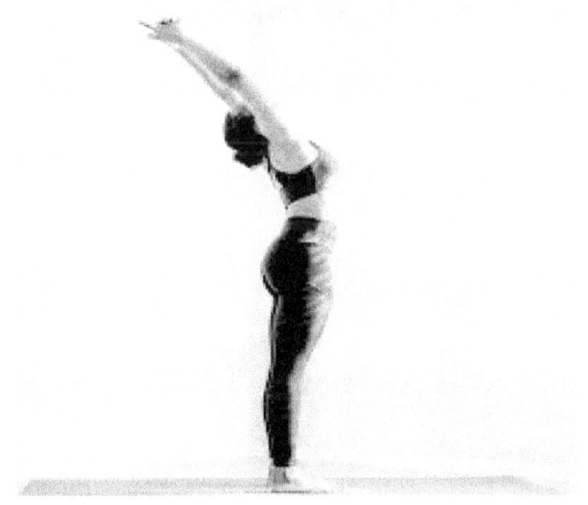

3. Slowly lean forward, hands touch the ground respectfully, head meets knees.

Breathing: Exhale

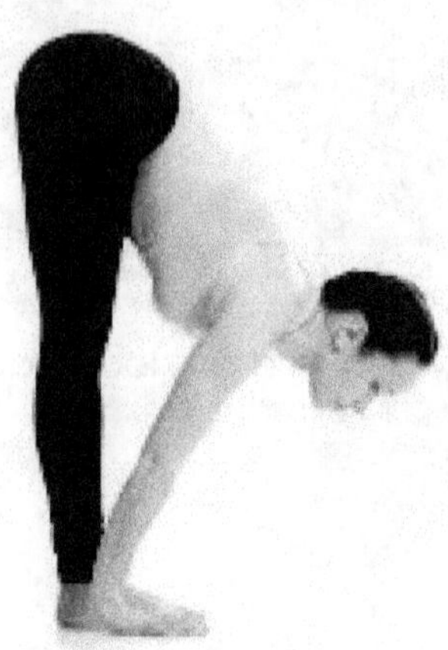

4. Place both hands firmly on the ground with the palms down, bring back the left knee, raise the head facing the Sun, hold maximum weight on the two palms, and ten fingers.

Breathing: Breath in

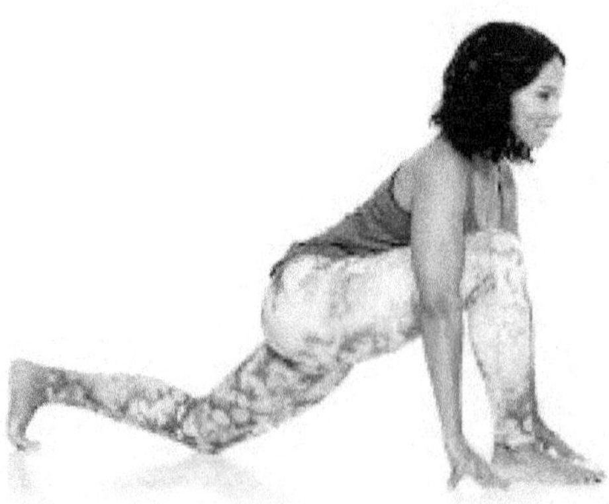

5. Take your right leg back next to your left leg, keep your hands and legs straight, bend your body to the hip forming an arch, just like a mountain, known as 'parvathasan' or mountain pose.'

Breathing: Exhale

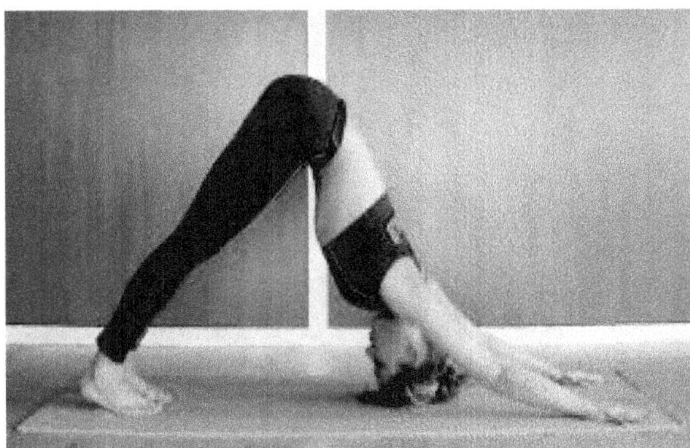

6. In the Namaskar Saashtanga pose, spread yourself fully to the ground (all eight 'anga' or body parts on the ground – head, leg, eyes (sight), face, word, feet, hands, and ears (hearing)). Feet, knees, thighs, shoulders, forehead touch the ground with hands stretched out and folded in place, with your mind and thoughts on the full namaskar, then turn the head slowly towards the sides first to the left and then to thc right so that each ear touches the ground.

Breathing: First inhale, and then completely exhale.

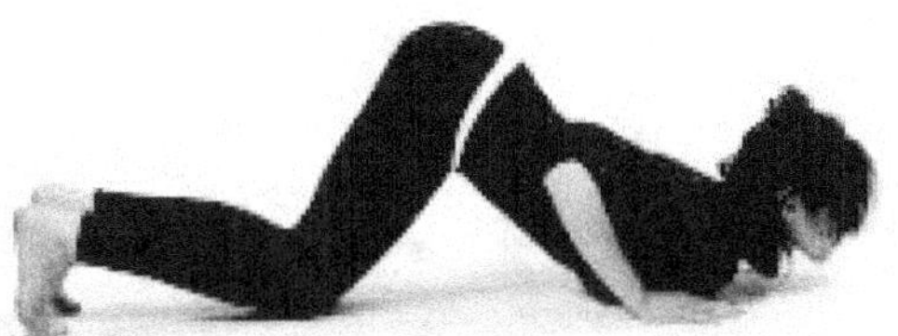

7. Head up slowly, bend as far back as possible, hands straight, in the cobra pose.

Breathing: Breathing in

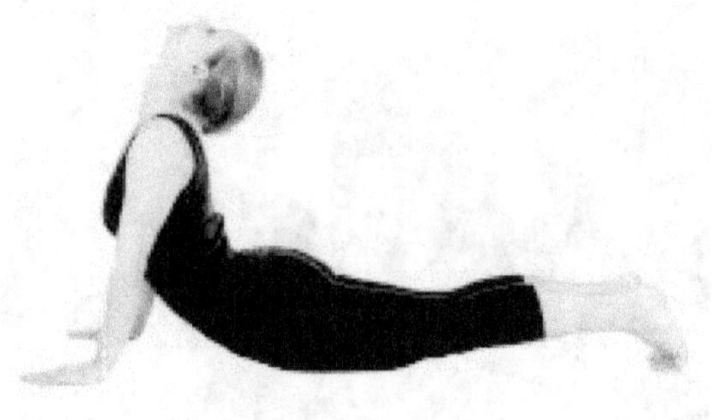

8. Parvathasan-just likes Step 5.

Breathing: Exhale

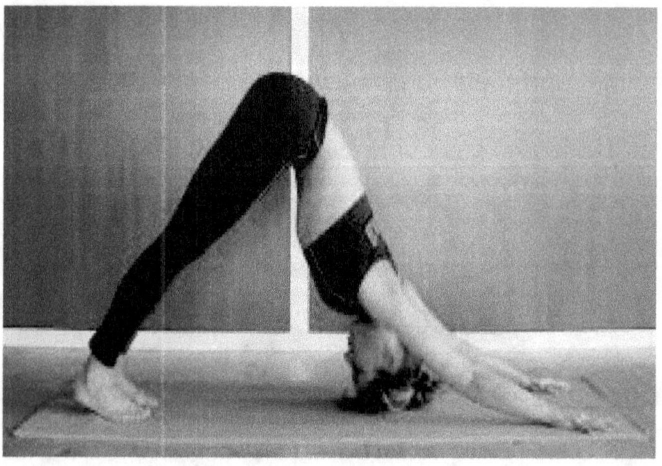

9. Same as Step 4, except for bringing the right leg forward.

Breathing: Breath in

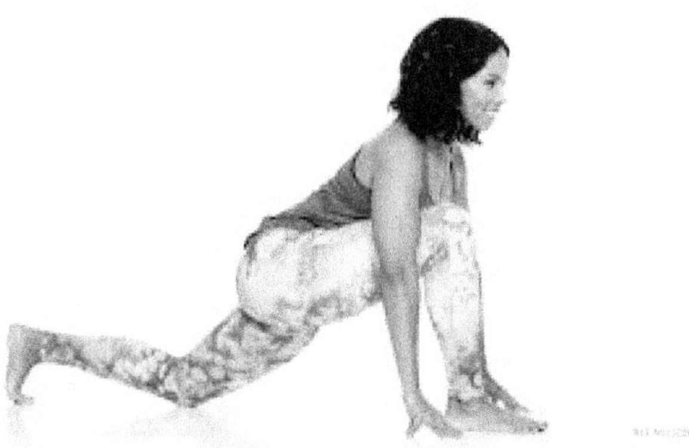

10. Like Step 3

Breathing: Exhale

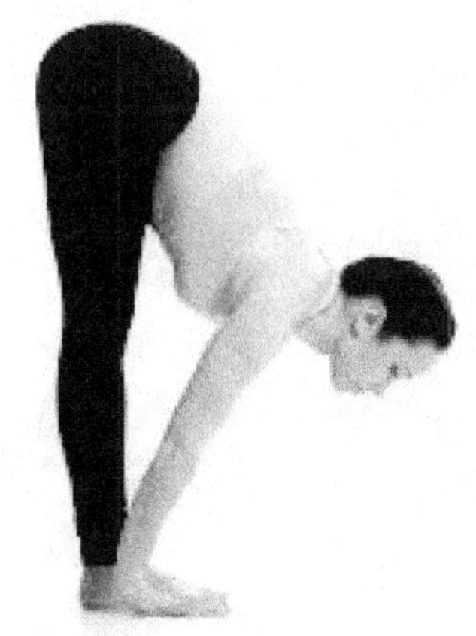

11. Like Step 2

Breathing: Breath in

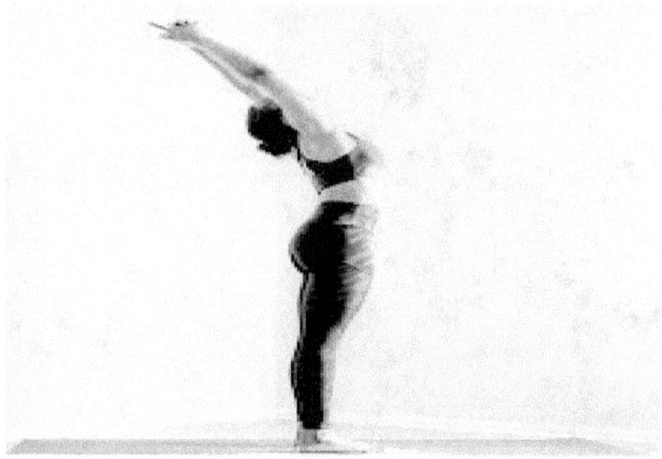

12. Like Step 1

Breathing: Exhale, inhale, and exhale.

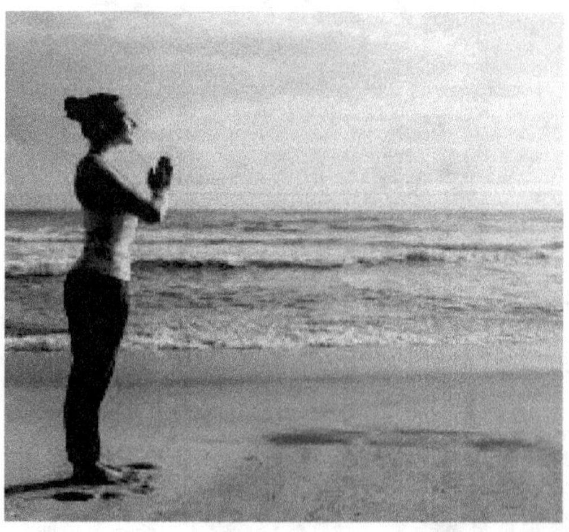

INTRODUCTION TO BANDHAS AND KRIYAS

Introduction to Bandha

Historically recognized as part of mudras, Bandhas were passed down by word of mouth from guru to disciple. The Hatha Yoga Pradipika deals with bandhas and mudras together, and the ancient tantric texts do not differentiate between the two. Bandhas are extensively incorporated throughout the mudra, as are the pranayama techniques. And their locking behaviour shows them as a deeply important group of activities, in their own right.

The Sanskrit word bandha means "holding,""tightening," or "locking." Such explanations accurately explain the bandha's physical activity and its effect on the pranic body. The bandhas intend to lock up the pranas in some areas and channel their flow into Sushumna nadi for purposes of spiritual awakening. Bandhas may be done separately or combined with mudra and pranayama practice. If the mental capacities are combined in this way they are awakened and form an alternative to higher yogic practice.

JALANDHARA BANDHA

Jalandhara Bandha (throat lock)

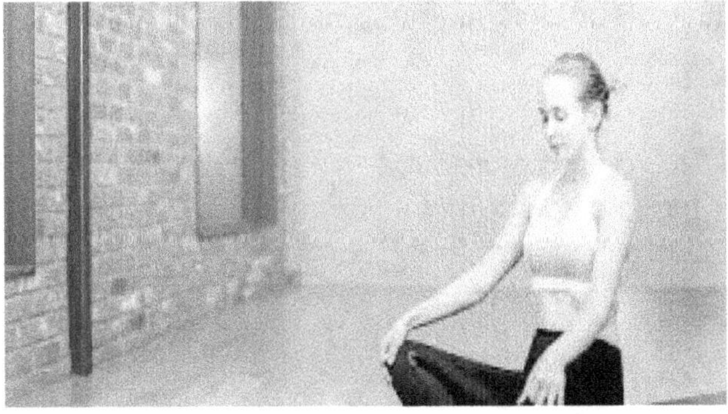

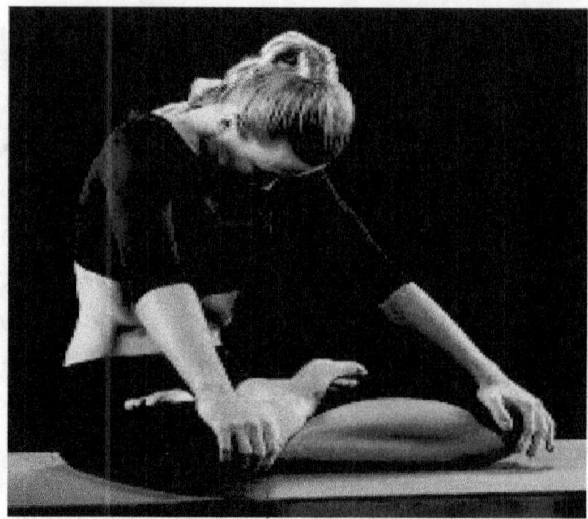

Rest in padmasana or Siddha / Siddha yoni asana straight with the head and spine The knees should be firmly in contact with the stone. Those who are unable to do this could be in a standing position performing bandha jalandhara. Place the palms of your hands on your knees. Close your eyes, and relax the whole body. Inhale deeply and steadily, then keep in the breath. Bend your head forward while holding your breath, and press the cheek tightly against the throat. Straighten the arms and firmly lock them in place, pushing down the knees with hands-on.

Hunch the head up and down, simultaneously. It will ensure that the weapons stay locked so the pressure applied to the back is increased. Stay at the final spot, as long as you can keep your breath comfortably. Don't put on the pressure. Relax the back, raise the jaw, progressively open the lock, lift the head and then exhale. Repeat until breathing is back to normal.

Variation: In kriya yoga, a more subtle sort of jalandhara bandha is done where the head is bent forward so the chin pushes the neck and the consciousness is centred on the vishuddhi chakra. This variant of the kriya is the most widely used in connection with practices of asana.

Breathing: The treatment can also be achieved with external oxygen retention.

Duration: Jalandhara bandha should be maintained for as long as the practitioner can keep the breath safe. Over this time maintaining a count slowly while retaining the width and rising the number one by one. The practice can be repeated up to 5 times.

Awareness: Visual-to mouth trap. Spiritual-on the vishuddhi Chakra.

Sequence: This bandha is ideally completed along with pranayamas and mudras. This should be performed after asanas and pranayamas, and, if practised alone, before meditation.

Contra-indications: The practice of Jalandhar bandha does not include people with cervical spondylosis, high intracranial pressure, vertigo, high blood pressure or heart disease. Although it initially reduces blood pressure, it induces some strain to the heart from long breath-hold.

Benefits: Jalandhara bandha compress the carotid sinuses on the carotid arteries, the neck's principal arteries. These sinuses help regulate the circulatory and respiratory systems. A reduction in oxygen and an increase of carbon dioxide in the body typically lead to higher heart rate and rapid respiration. The loop is triggered by the carotid sinuses.

This tendency is avoided by exerting artificial pressure on these sinuses, allowing a reduced heart rate and improved breath retention. This practice provides mental stimulation, calming stress, anxiety and anger. In meditation, this causes introversion and one-pointedness. The stimulation of the throat helps in controlling thyroid function and in regulating metabolism.

Practice Note: Do not inhale or exhale until the chin lock is locked and the armlock is removed. If the feeling of suffocation is felt then immediately pause and relax. If the feeling has passed the procedure continues.

Note: The Sanskrit word Jalan means net and Dhara means the current or flux. One understanding of the Jalandhar bandha is the lock within the neck that regulates the nadis network. The real representation of these nadis is the blood vessels and the neck nerves. An alternate interpretation is that it would mean 'throat, Jalan, water' and Dhara refers to a tubular vessel in the body. Hence, Jalandhara bandha is the throat lock that protects the nectar or fluid that flows down from Bindu to vishuddhi and prevents it from falling into the digestive stream.

That way, prana is conserved. There's a different view, too. Adhara means 'substrate' or 'foundation.' The body has seventeen separate centres called adharas that refer to the chakras of major and minor significance. Jalandhara bandha can also be defined as the practice of locking the pranic network of the neck and redirecting the flow of subtle energy from adhering to the Sushumna nadi of the spine.

MOOLA BANDHA

The technique I: Moola Bandha (perineum contraction)

Phase I: To apply pressure to the perineal/vaginal region, sit in Siddha / Siddha yoni asana. Close your eyes, let your whole body relax. Be aware of the natural environment for a short moment. Then the sensitivity focuses on the perineal/vaginal region. Secure this region by drawing muscles on the pelvic floor and then relaxing them. Continue to contract slightly, and relax the perineal/vaginal area as rhythmically and consistently as possible.

Phase 2: Gradually contract this region, and keep the contraction going. Continue breathing normally; do not hold breath. Be completely conscious of what the sensation is. Stretch out a little further but keep the rest of the body relaxed. Just contact those muscles which are connected to the mooladhara area. The anal and urinary sphincters are still contracting in the beginning, but this will be reduced and will eventually cease as greater sensitivity and control is developed. Ultimately the practitioner encounters one point of movement towards the foot. Relax the muscles slowly, and uniformly. Place the tension on the spine to help focus on the point of contracture. 10 times repeat with total contracture and absolute relaxation.

Technique 2: Moola Bandha with internal breath retention

Sit in an asana pose in which the feet firmly meet the floor. Siddha / Siddha yoni asana or moola bandhasana are the best asanas which move the heel into the perineum and help improve the performance of the bandha. Place your hands on your thighs. Close your eyes, and relax over the entire body for a few minutes. Hold the air in, inhale deeply and perform bandha jalandhara. Perform moola bandha by progressively contracting the perineal/vaginal region and maintaining as strong a contraction as possible. Don't put on the pressure. The above lock is this. Keep on for as long as you can safely carry the oxygen. Slowly release bandha moola, raise the head upright, and exhale. Up to 10 practice times.

Breathing: The process above can also be done with an external oxygen chain.

Consciousness: When taking the final position and performing jalandhara bandha, physical consciousness should be focused on the air. At the place of perineal contraction, the consciousness should be placed in the final position. Spiritual-at breath, and then on mooladhara chakra during contraction.

Contra-indications: Only an experienced yoga instructor can perform this exercise. Moola bandha increases energy very quickly, which may precipitate hyperactivity symptoms if performed improperly or if there is no comprehensive preparation.

Benefits: The bandha Moola has many physical, emotional, and spiritual benefits. The pelvic nerves are stimulated, toning up the urogenital and excretory structures. The intestinal peristalsis is also triggered, which relieves constipation and the piles. Sometimes helpful are anal fissures, ulcers, prostatitis, multiple types of prostatic hypertrophy and recurrent pelvic infections. As this action releases steam, this is also useful in the treatment of psychosomatic and some degenerative disorders.

The effects spread through the brain and endocrine system across the body making it especially beneficial in cases of asthma, bronchitis and arthritis. This also calms down on depression. The quality of this activity leads to a spontaneous realignment of the physical, emotional, and psychic bodies in preparation for spiritual awakening. Moola bandha is both a way to gain sexual regulation (brahmacharya) and to alleviate many sexual disorders. This makes either the upward movement of sexual energy for spiritual growth or downward movement to enhance marital ties. This helps to alleviate the feelings of sexual discomfort, repression of sexual desire and sexual guilt.

Practice note: Moola bandha is the contraction of some muscles in the pelvic floor. The entire perineum does not contract. In the male body, the area of contraction lies between the anus and the testes. In the female body, the point of contracture is behind the cervix, where the uterus reaches into the vagina. It's the subtle-level energizing of the mooladhara chakra. The perineal body, which is the convergence point of several muscles inside the groin, acts as a trigger point for the location of the mooladhara chakra. These areas are initially difficult to separate, and it is recommended that Ashwini and vajroli mudras be mastered first in preparation for moola bandha.

Note: The Sanskrit word moola means 'root,' 'firmly set,' 'source' or 'trigger.' In this sense, it refers to the root of the spine or the perineum where the mooladhara chakra, the location of the kundalini, the primal power, is located. Moola bandha stimulates Brahma granthi efficiently and locates and awakens the chakra of mooladhara.

UDDIYANA BANDHA

Preparatory practice: Standing abdominal contraction

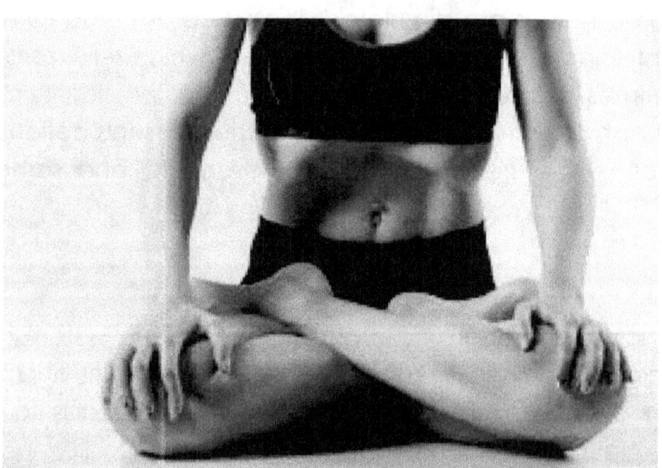

Stand upright with feet about half a meter apart. Inhale deeply, through the nostrils. Bend in from the knees and exhale all the air through the mouth. Start emptying as many of the lungs as possible. Keep your neck straight, and bend your elbows slightly. Place the palms of the hand on the thighs just above the knees, so that knees support the upper body weight. The fingers may point either downwards, or one to the other.

Make sure your arms remain straight. In this place the abdominal region contracts immediately. Attach the chin to the chest then lean the head forward. Keep the glottis closed, make a fake inhalation and open the throat as if breathing in but not taking in air. Straighten the legs up slightly. This motion will immediately pull the abdomen upwards and inwards towards the spine to form uddiyana bandha. Keep a good time at this venue. Don't put on the pressure. Remove the abdominal lock, and let the throat relax. Straighten the feet, and raise the chin. Exhale slowly to ease the pressure on the lungs and then gradually breathe in through the nose. Keep standing until breathing gets back to normal before the next round begins.

Uddiyana Bandha (abdominal contraction)

Sit in Siddha / Siddha yoni asana or padmasana with the spine upright and legs in contact with the floor. Padding can be used for raising the thighs, lowering the knees. Place the palms of your hands flat on your knees. Close your eyes, let your whole body relax. Inhale from the nostrils, deeply. Exhale through the mouth with a whoosh, then empty as much of the lungs as possible. Keep the gas out. Step forward and bring palms of your hand down on the thighs. Straighten the elbows and raise arms, allowing further stretch of the spinal cord.

Randomly do jalandhara bandha, pressing the chin against the side. Drive the abdominal muscles inwards and outwards. Keep out the abdominal lock and relax, without straining, as long as possible. Then release the bolt, bend the elbows and drop the shoulders to the abdomen. Head down, and then slowly inhale. Stay in that position until the breath returns to normal, and then start the next round.

Breathing: Uddiyana bandha is only done by maintaining external oxygen.

Duration: Initially practice 3 rounds and progressively increase over a few months to 10 rounds as the machine becomes accustomed to the practice.

Awareness: Physical-on the abdomen and synchronizing the breath with each step. Spiritual-on the Manipura chakra.

Sequence: Uddiyana bandha is simpler to do if followed by an inverted asana.

Precaution: Uddiyana bandha is an advanced technique and can only be tried on instruction after learning some skills in breath-holding, as well as jalandhara and moola bandhas.

Contra-indications: People with colitis, stomach or intestinal ulcer, diaphragm hernia, elevated blood pressure, heart disease, glaucoma and increased intracranial pressure should not take this treatment. Even it can be stopped by pregnant women.

Benefits: Uddiyana bandha is the panacea for many abdominal and stomach issues, including constipation, indigestion, worms, and diabetes, unless they're chronic. It stimulates digestive fire, and it massages and tones the abdominal organs. It controls the adrenal glands, reducing lethargy and relaxing stress and anxiety. This increases blood flow to the entire body region and protects all internal organs.

Uddiyana bandha stimulates the solar plexus which has several subtle effects on the distribution of body-wide energy. This creates a suction pressure that reverses the flow of the sub-pranas, Apana, and prana, uniting them to Samana and stimulating Manipura chakra. Then there is an explosion of subtle force which moves upwards through Sushumna nadi.

Practice note: Uddiyana bandha should always be done on an empty stomach, as well as cleaning the intestines. Agnisar kriya is an excellent training course.

Note: The Sanskrit word uddiyana means "rising" or "moving up," as the physical lock applied to the body causes the diaphragm to rise to the throat. So Uddiyana is also translated as stomach uplifting. Another meaning is that the physical lock helps direct prana into Sushumna nadi so that it can flow up into the Sahasrara chakra.

Kriya yoga offers a unique approach

Kriya yoga means 'practice, movement, or action yoga.' Unlike the many religious, philosophical, or yogic practices that involve mental discipline, the key advice in the kriya yoga system is, 'Do not worry about the mind.' If your mind is dissipating or there are disruptions in your mind and you cannot even focus for a second, that doesn't matter. You just need to carry on with your activities as you can still evolve, even without questioning, controlling or trying to control the mind.

This is a new concept of human life and most people certainly have never even considered it.

The first thing they are taught is to control the mind when taking to religion, beginning spiritual practices, or going to gurus. 'And you might suggest it. And you don't think so. Only something you have to do. Do not. This is completely fine. That is bad. That is bad. Do not sin.' And so on. Many conclude that the mind is the divine existence's greatest barrier, but that is a very misguided and risky notion. The mind is a bridge between this and that, so how could that be a barrier? A fool believes this is an obstacle and tries to break the bridge. Instead, after he has lost it, he wonders how to get to the other side. It is the unfortunate fate of most people and it is, unfortunately, the religions, principles and values that are responsible for it. People who are less mindful of morality and ethics don't have mental disorders. We are simply healthy, happy-go-lucky people.

TEACHING METHODOLOGY ON BANDHAS AND KRIYAS

BANDHAS

BASIC TECHNIQUES

1. Mula Bandha

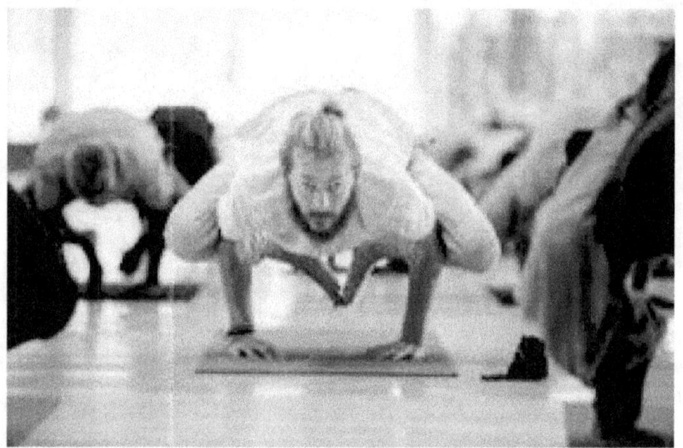

Use left-hand heel to press the Yoni. Maintain the right heel pressed over the area just above the heart of the neck. Contract the anus, and compile the Apana Vayu. Mula Bandha is named after him. The Apana Vayu which performs the role of excreting ejection has a natural tendency to move downward. Via the guidance of Mula Bandha, the Apana Vayu is made to shift upward by contracting the anus and pushing it upward aggressively. The Prana Vayu is merged with the Apana and permitted by the unified Prana-Apana Vayu to join the Sushumna Nadi. And the yogi attains perfection in Yoga. Kundalini is confused.

The Yogi drinks the Necktar of Life. He in Chakra Sahasrara loves Siva-pada. He is all sanctified by Vibhutis and Aishvarya. If the Apana is joined to Prana, Anahata's sounds (mystical inner tones) are heard very clearly. Enter Prana, Apana, Nada and Bindu in Yoga, and attain perfection through the Yogi. The highest point can not be reached by the first attempt. One can do this again and again for a long time. The

Siddhi is achieved in pranayama practice with the aid of Bandhas and Mudras. The practise of Mula Bandha helps one to hold full Brahmacharya, provides Dhatu-Pushti (nerve-vigour), relieves constipation and increases Jatharagni. Mula Bandha can be combined with all other Yogic Kriyas in the practice of concentration, meditation, pranayama.

2. Jalandhara Bandha

Contract back. The head is pushed stiffly against the stomach. This Bandha is done at the end of Puraka and beginning of Kumbhaka. Usually, this Bandha is done during the Kumbhaka only. The gastric fire, located in the Nabhi region, absorbs the nectar from the Sahasrara Chakra which exudes through the hole in the palate. Hence this Bandha prevents nectar ingestion.

3. Uddiyana Bandha

The Sanskrit word 'Uddiyana' comes from the root 'ut' and 'di' which means 'go up.' When this Bandha is done the Prana flies up through the Sushumna Nadi. So that's the notable name. Clear the lungs by an efficient and forcible expiration. If you exhale from your mouth vigorously the lungs get empty. Now push and move the intestines towards the back over and under the navel, so the abdomen lies high up in the thoracic cavity towards the back of the body. That is Uddiyana Bandha. This is achieved at the end of Kumbhaka and beginning of Rechaka.

The diaphragm, the muscle segment between the abdomen and the thoracic cavity, is raised and the abdominal muscles are drawn backwards while you perform this Bandha. The exercise can be performed with ease as you bend your trunk forward. Uddiyana Bandha is the very first statement that Nauli Kriya makes. You should know Uddiyana Bandha if you wish to perform the Nauli Kriya.

The Nauli Kriya is usually performed in a standing position. Uddiyana Bandha can be done in a sitting or standing posture. Place your hands onto the thigh as seen in the illustration while standing. This exercise does everything to help Brahmacharya stay awake. It endows beautiful fitness, strength, vigour and vitality to the practitioner. When combined with Nauli Kriya it serves as a potent gastrointestinal tonic. They are the two powerful instruments of the Yogin to counter constipation, poor peristalsis of the bowel and other disorders of the food channel. It is through these two Yogic Kriyas alone that it is possible to monitor and relax all abdominal muscles. For abdominal exercises, nothing can challenge Uddiyana Bandha and Nauli. We remain unique across all physical activity programs and unrivalled. Uddiyana and Nauli performed a fast, thorough, and wonderful cure in chronic diseases of the stomach and intestines where all kinds of drugs have failed.

When you practice the Pranayama, you can beautifully combine Mula Bandha, Jalandhara Bandha, and Uddiyana Bandha. It is Bandha-Traya. Uddiyana Bandha does away with abdominal fat. In cases where the Marienbud reduction pills have failed to reduce fat, Uddiyana Bandha may work wonders. They can do Uddiyana if fatty people avoid taking ghee and reduce drinking water. A foot trip to Kedar-Badri or Mount Kailas will bring fatty people into the practice of Uddiyana Bandha.

KRIYA

BASIC TECHNIQUES

Talabya Kriya

The kriyaban sticks the tongue to the palate starting from a relaxed stance, creating an effect of a suction cup and holding the tip of the tongue always turned towards the teeth. Someone opens the mouth so that it can be shut off by the tongue, which has been connected to the palate for a few instants; the stretching effect on the Fraenulum tongue can be felt. Pulling the tongue straight out of the mouth. It replicates this work 50 times [initially no more than 10 times!]. After months of practice, this technique produces the Kechari Mudra: inserting the tongue into the nasal pharynx cavity, keeping it firmly in that position with a physical and mental effort-initially with the help of one or two fingers pushing the tongue close to its root. [Lahiri Mahasaya strongly opposed cutting Fraenulum to get faster and simpler results].

Most people perform the Talabya Kriya incorrectly because they automatically turn their tongue backwards (or keep it upright), erasing the whole effect. To meet the teeth the tongue must continue pointing outward until it sticks to the palate. This technique has a perceptible calming impact on the mechanism of thinking; hence, it can never be left aside before the Kechari Mudra is attained. It's unclear why this activity on the Fraenulum will reduce thinking growth. Nevertheless, by simply practising it, everyone can easily verify the calming effect of Talabya Kriya. [Note. Talabya Kriya's effect is intensified by the following exercises: dragging the tongue past the nose tip with the aid of a piece of cloth around it. Then follow using an index or middle finger to move the tongue back.]

Navi Kriya

By attempting to control the breath, one's consciousness travels slowly along the spinal column, placing the syllable Om [ooooong] in the first five chakras, and even in Kutastha, skipping the sixth chakra. The head is turned down towards the chest and Om is whispered in the navel about 75 times [one may use beads to hold the count, but a rough approximation is fine], either verbally or mentally-. The hands are cross-fingered together with the palms downwards; the thumbs strike the navel at very gentle pressure for each single Om.

The head is then raised [to a limited degree, but as much as possible, feeling muscle tension at the base of the neck], the mind drifts first to Bindu and then down to the third Chakra. Om is chanted-in the third chakra, either verbally or mentally-about 25 times. The hands are positioned with the palms upwards and the fingers crossed behind the back, and the thumbs exert gentle pressure on the lumbar vertebrae with each Om. [Breath is not associated with Om singing, by all means.]

The chin's normal position is then restored, and the Om is believed to be in every Chakra, from Kutastha to Muladhara. This is one complete cycle of the Navi Kriya. One shouldn't skip doing at least 4 cycles of Navi Kriya. When we go along with the practice, calm energy is considered to collect in the centre of the Samana current, in the middle-lower portion of the abdomen.

ASANAS TOBALANCE THE HEALTH AND ITS YOGIC VIEW

In Patanjali's Yoga Sutras, a descriptive definition of yogasanas is given: "Sthiramsukhamaasanam," meaning 'the comfortable and stable position.' In this sense, asanas are performed to cultivate the ability to sit comfortably in one position for an extended period, a skill required for meditation. Raja yoga is the yogasana equivalent of a balanced sitting. The Hatha yogis, however, find that such particular body positions, asanas, open the energy channels and the mental centres. They noticed that learning body control, through these activities, helped them to regulate mind and energy.

Yogasanas became instruments for greater awareness, providing the secure foundation necessary for the exploration of the body, air, mind, and higher states. For this reason, asana practice comes first in hatha yoga texts such as Hatha Yoga Pradipika. In the yogic scriptures, it is said that there were originally 8,400,000 asanas, representing the 8,400,000 incarnations that each person must pass through before they attain liberation from the life and death cycles. These asanas reflected a gradual progression from the simplest form of life to the most complex: that of a fully developed human being. Over the years the great rishis and yogis modified and decreased the number of asanas to the few hundred known today. By their practice, it is possible to side-step the karmic cycle and to skip several developmental stages in one lifetime. Of those few hundred, only the eighty-four most important are addressed in depth.

Yogasanas and prana

Prana, an integral force that correlates to ki or chi in Chinese medicine, pervades the whole body, following flow patterns, called nadis, which are responsible for controlling all individual cellular activity. Body stiffness is due to blocked prana, and subsequent accumulation of toxins. If prana starts flowing, the toxins are removed from the system which ensures the health of the whole body. As the body is supple, postures that seemed impossible are easier to perform and it develops steadiness and grace of movement. If the amount of prana is increased to a great extent, the body shifts into other postures by itself, and asanas, mudras, and pranayamas naturally occur.

Yogasanas and kundalini

The ultimate aim of yoga is to awaken the kundalini shakti, in the capacity of man for evolution. The practice of asanas stimulates the chakras, distributing the kundalini energy that is generated throughout the body. For this reason, approximately 35 asanas are explicitly planned: bhujangasana for Manipura chakra, Sarvangasana for vishuddhi, Sirshasana for Sahasrara, etc. The other asanas regulate and purify the body's nadis, allowing for prana conduction. The main aim of hatha yoga is to strike a balance between the mental and pranic powers that interfere with activities and processes. The impulses generated when this has been accomplished give Sushumna nadi, the central pathway in the spine through which the kundalini shakti ascends to the Sahasrara chakra, illuminating the higher centres of human consciousness, a call to awakening. Hatha yoga therefore not only strengthens the body and enhances health but also activates and awakens the higher centres responsible for the development of human consciousness.

Yogasanas and the body-mind connection

Mind and body are not distinct entities though they can think and behave as though they were. In the body and mind, the gross mental form is the subtle body shape. Practice Asana embeds and harmonizes them. Body harbour tensions or knots as well as mind harbour. Every mental knot has its physiological, physical knot and vice versa. Asana is working at loosening certain knots. Asanas reduce mental burdens to the mind through the body when engaging with them on the physical level, behaving somato-psychically.

For example, emotional stresses and agitation can strain and obstruct the smooth functioning of the lungs, diaphragm, and respiration system, leading to a very disabled asthma-like disease. Muscle knots can occur anywhere in the body: tightness of the neck as cervical spondylitis, facial as neuralgia, etc. A well-selected series of asanas, along with pranayama, shatkarmas, meditation and Nidra yoga, is most effective in resolving these knots and overcoming them from both the mental and physical levels. The result is that latent energy is released; the body becomes full of vitality and strength; and the mind becomes vibrant, creative, happy, and healthy.

ADJUSTING AND ASSISTING YOGA ASANA

The Heart of Practicing and Guiding Yoga

We all start from where we are when practising yoga at the risk of saying the obvious — this in contrast to where anyone else may think we are or where we might mistakenly think we are ourselves. Most teachers have preconceived or misinformed ideas about the abilities or desires of their students, and many students overestimate or underestimate their capacity to immediately be present. How do we, as students, better cope with those conditions? By encouraging our students to develop a personal practice that reflects their values, priorities, and circumstances, as well as all those that grow (and are likely to). Several basic elements are ideally communicated to our students in each lesson and given even greater clarification to newer students. Among the most notable is the assumption that yoga is neither a comparative nor competitive practice, despite some people doing their best to make it that way.

It will make the profession healthier, more effective and more transformative to pursue this simple sensibility. It is a sensitivity — a fundamental yogic value — that reflects the sole comment on asana found in the often-cited Yoga Sutras of Patanjali: sthira, sukham, asana — meaning steadfastness, ease, and presence of mind (the latter, from the root word as, meaning "to take one seat," which I interpret as meaning to be here now, totally attuned to one's immediate experience). Relating to these is advantageous as values which we are still cultivating. Recall that Patanjali may not even describe anything slightly approximating the kind of postural practices that began to evolve several hundred years later and eventually became Hatha Yoga, which evolved more in the past seventy-five years than in the preceding thousand.

Crossing the Bridge from Practicing to Guiding

As we do yoga practice we come across different asanas. We are already experiencing sensations in approaching them. If we practice yoga rather than just running then we consciously breathe and use the air to refine how we learn asana. When consciously breathing, we bring more conscious consciousness into the body's mind, ideally as demonstrated by the momentary stimulus, changing our posture and positioning to be more steady, relaxed and present. So there's a breath dance with the body-mind, each influencing the other, all of which is progressively felt like part of our whole being. This is the essential practice of always and forever convergence and awakening which is at the centre of the yoga asana practice. Through it, we will play with different breathing exercises, positions, and visualizations, exploring their various effects and the inner dialogue and responses that are an increasingly direct reflection of our deeper qualities of being.

Guiding with Your Hands

By using your hands to accentuate and reinforce what you're trying to convey in words or visual images, a student's ability to understand and internalize what you're trying to say can make all the difference. (When dealing with hands-on adjustments, motivation, support, touch and so on, we use hands-on in both the general and the particular sense of the word — a general reference to physical guidance that may involve the use of one's hands, arms, shoulders, stomach, thighs, legs or feet, and a specific reference to one's hands.

Therefore touch, which explicitly and personally reaches our students immediately, can be an effective way to communicate explicitly, simply and precisely with them. Speaking words and physical presentation of asanas are important ways of communicating with students and should be the starting point for teaching asanas — and also the stopping point. But when combined with precise and knowledgeable touches these approaches will convey even more:

• Explain verbalized or confirmed alignment cue

• Physical activity to be emphasized

• Make students feel comfortable

• Feeling an unconscious portion of the body

• Helps stabilize, relax, or deepen asana

• Helping to safely expand motion range

• Helping you as a teacher become more conscious of the general state of the student

• Build a more positive and open sense of interaction between you and your students • Provide confidence in the strength of such experiences

INTRODUCTION TO YOGA ANATOMY

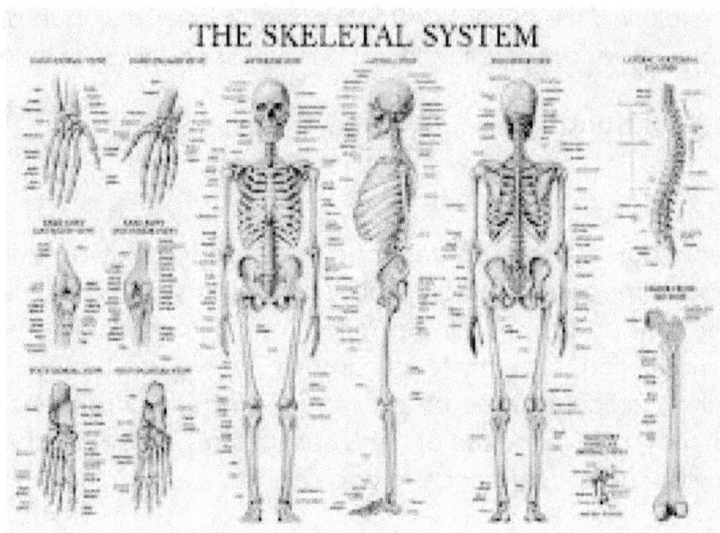

The human body is the platform in which to view the world and our physical yoga practice. Physical processes – the nervous, digestive, endocrine, and circulatory systems, and so on – serve as a barometer for this experience. For example, as a result of daily yoga practice, you can remember the ability to remain calm, to maintain space between yourself and stressful situations. Stress hormones become less nervous, as yoga and meditation's soothing effects keep the nerves relaxed.

The musculoskeletal system responds to exercise in many ways. Thanks to asana's relaxing effects you experience less back pain from it. When ranges of movement increase across the shoulders and chest, the capacity to take a complete breath of air increases, and the frequency of pain in the shoulder and neck decreases. A greater sense of well-being, peace of mind, and a lack of distraction from pain can very well lead to a more truthful and enjoyable view of life. Understanding the workings of the body offers a basis for passing on the body's experience to others. By enhancing your fluency in realistic, physical anatomy, it improves your eloquence and creativity as a Yoga teacher. Professional teaching blends the science and the craft. This section includes a brief description of the musculoskeletal system as it applies to movement in both functional and asana. A basic understanding of functional anatomy will help you as a teacher orchestrate a creative, enjoyable, and effective yoga class.

POWER OF MIND AND EIGHT FOLDS OF YOGA

Patanjali's Classical Yoga refers to the "Eight-Limbed Path" yoga practice. Like a tree with various branches branching from the same trunk, the eight limbs are different forms of practice that lead to the same goal of the reunification of Consciousness. The knowledge with which we seek communion is our true existence, as an embodied spirit. Although the depiction of branches on a tree implies a sequential approach the limbs may operate at the same time to bring us closer to our basic nature. A detailed explanation can be found in B.K.S. Iyengar's "Light on Yoga." The extremities are:

Yamas- ethical disciplines

Niyamas- self-observation

Asana- Posture

Pranayama -Life energy participation through breath

Pratyahara - Sensory withdrawal

Dharana- Concentration

Dhyana- Meditation

Samadhi- Highest Consciousness Recognition

Yamas

The Yamas are fundamental ethical concepts that refer to values that endorse the practice of yoga and encourage meditation: non-violence, truthfulness, non-stealing, self-restraint, and non-hardiness. A spontaneous non-violent activity represents an understanding that we are all connected to every human being. What we do for anyone else we do for ourselves, as we are both facets of the Same.

Niyamas

Niyamas are individual disciplines which include purity, contentment, involvement, self-study and devotion. Within the Yogi these qualities can be developed — maybe a better word would be "revealed." One might think of all the Yamas and Niyamas as disciplines that display our true nature. Continuous effort and dedication are therefore necessary because otherwise our unconscious habits and predilections will remain unseen.

Asana

Asana practice encourages physical strength, endurance, agility, a balanced nervous system, and the ability to sit for periods without pain which is a required prerequisite for meditation. Patanjali in his Yoga Sutras refers only to asana as a pose for meditation and probably has never foreseen the present focus as part of asana practice on physical ability and fashion.

Each of us is a little different in physicality, bone structure and affinity for the aspects of yoga practice. Many of us won't be able to sit in meditation because the body's energies are scattered at first, and one-pointed concentration is difficult. Practice mindful asana creates a physical and balanced body capable of withdrawing into itself because performing postures is an activity of actively moving prana. Without this knowledge, yoga practice will not be able to "heal the body of the restlessness that is a sign of its incapacity to absorb the vital forces poured into it from the universal Life-Ocean without working them out in action and motion" (Sri Aurobindo).

Pranayama

Not just breath-control, pranayama. Prana is responsible for all of the body's functions — heart, lungs, brain, and air, or vital life-force. The breath is our clearest relationship to prana and the one we can most influence on. Practising pranayama brings us one step closer to enhancing our understanding of the prana movement within ourselves. It is not to approach the task of being more open with an attitude of dominance, strength or resilience, but rather an opportunity to lay the ego aside and consider it.

Pratyahara

When the body becomes even more ready and the prana movement becomes apparent, the elimination of senses becomes practicable. This practice stage is similar to ripples quieting on a lake. External objects are seen as temporary only, whether they want the mind to create or something else. When we no longer cling to these objects and non-attachment becomes possible our true nature turns inward.

Dharana

Dharana is a highly centred state, stable with prana movement. The condition is a pathway to meditation.

Dyana

This is the deep trance state in which the Yogi is fully absorbed and the senses are stilled in. The lake of human consciousness is so still that it reflects the real reality, that everything is One.

Samadhi

Classical Yoga states here that individual experience blends with the collective consciousness. It is said that the happiness that we feel here is millions of times that of the real, separate mind. Bliss, in this situation, is beyond ordinary knowledge and any words.

CORE YOGA FOR BETTER DIGESTION

There are twelve pairs of ribs: the upper seven ribs are the actual ribs, while the 8th, 9th, and 10th ribs are the false ribs, and the floating ribs are the 11th and 12th ribs. Both the ribs interact with the thoracic vertebrae. The parts of the cartilage of actual ribs articulate with the sternum. The cartilage portions of the false ribs are attached and the cartilage part of the seventh rib is attached, thereby being indirectly connected to the sternum. The floating ribs are without contact. The cartilage parts of the ribs are sensitive for thorax elasticity, and thus it is important to stretch the transverse thoracic muscle that links the sternum with the ribs. The ribs move precisely with each breath.

With the inhalation, the upper two ribs pass forward and back, while the lower ribs turn outwards, while the middle ribs merge both motions. The upper sternum goes back and forth, and the lower sternum goes farther backwards. During exhalation, certain movements are passively reversed. The basic exercises were chosen to coordinate all of those processes. The assisted bending exercises stretch the intercostal muscles forward, backwards and especially to the sides and improve joint mobility with the ribs. Even the front of the upper thorax must be stretched, as it is too short in many cases.

It is necessary to maintain a neutral lumbopelvic posture to target the motions directly at the ribs. The elasticity of the thorax and the effectiveness of breathing can be maintained with age or even increased. More alveoli which also grow in the lungs as the thorax is expanded. This raises the surface area for exchanging oxygen and carbon dioxide, leading to improved supply of oxygen to all body systems.

Experiencing the Abdominals as Stabilizers

Understanding how to use your abdominal muscles as stabilisers will improve your ability to practice asana while protecting your spine, especially your lower back. It will also make you feel more secure in your movements and help you eliminate some of the possible pressure that requires arm strength from your shoulders in asana, such as the Up-Plank Pose (Chaturanga Dandasana). In this section, we will talk about some simple exercises.

EXERCISE

Lifting the Head

TO EXPERIENCE THE ABDOMINAL MUSCLES AS STABILIZERS

CAUTIONS: Do not perform after eating the second portion of this workout, or if you have osteoporosis or other issues with your rib.

PROP: 1 mat with no skid

Part 1.

Lie down on the bunk, on the right. Place your arms one foot apart comfortably around your sides and back. To calm down, take a few breaths and get in the centre. Instead, keep your knees together until your kneecaps meet the ceiling. Place the navel one side over. Using an exhalation to raise your head off the floor, and remember what you feel under your hand. You'll no doubt feel the abdominal muscles contracting. Put your head down, and try again. This contraction is a good example of abdominal muscular stabilisation.

The muscles that generate your head's lifting movement are the flexors of the neck that are in the anterior, or front, arm. But the abdominal muscles are needed to make this move because the abdominals hold the rib cage still so that the neck flexors can do their job, which is to lift the head. What the abdominals do is direct the movement by keeping the rib cage still and allowing the flexor movement of the neck to do just that: Flex the neck against gravity. It'll be tough — maybe impossible — but try to lift your head off the floor without contracting your abdominals.

Place your hand over your navel and lift your head as the abdominal muscles relax. If you have a strong neuromuscular device that works well, it would certainly not be possible. This test makes it clear what happens to someone paralyzed from the shoulder downwards, and therefore unable to raise his head off the bed. He still has neurologically intact and functional neck flexor muscles, but because his abdominal muscles can not contract due to a lack of nerve control, thus stabilizing the rib cage, he faces severe difficulty when he tries to raise his head. The importance of abdominal muscles acting as a group to stabilize the trunk is difficult to overemphasise and will be explored in more detail as we go along.

LIFTING THE HEAD

Part 2.

Ask a friend to kneel by your stomach and face your eyes for a better understanding of how the abdominals function as stabilizers. When you exhale, your assist will press tightly down on your lower ribs so they drop into your chest for around 2 inches. Following the normal rib curve, her fingers will point outward and downward. A word of warning here: With this pressure, it should feel intense but not painful. Try to raise your head when she's pushed down and keep your ribs still. It should feel very good because the pressure from the hands increases the stability needed to the rib cage so that the neck flexors can do their job of raising the head. This exercise illustrates not only the strength of stabilization but also how abdominal muscles can help shape habits that occur in other areas of the body.

EXERCISE

Lifting One Leg

TO CREATE AWARENESS OF ABDOMINALSTABILIZATION

CAUTION: Do not exercise this during the last two trimesters of pregnancy.

PROP: 1 mat with no skid

Part 1.

Lie on your back mat, close your eyes and imagine elevating your right leg from the floor. Then just think about moving your knee but then don't move it: just remember what's going on. You'll probably feel multiple muscles contracting, among them the chief abdominals. Now, heave your right leg off the board. Notice that when you do this the abdominal contraction increases immensely. Drop your leg to the floor, and do the same with the other leg. Think about raising the knee first of all. But just bring your knee up. If you try to lift one leg you will find that it is much easier to keep your pelvis still than when you try to lift the other leg. If so, the opposite sides of the abdominal muscles are not equal in strength.

LIFTING ONE LEG

Part 2.

To make this exercise even harder, lift one leg about 5 inches off the floor, then move it outwards around 10 inches. If you find that your leg is moving a little externally while you are doing this, no problem: it's natural and it's linked to your hip joint. If your abdominal muscles balance your trunk full, so there will be no rolling of your pelvis there will be no uplifting of the opposite pelvis. Bring your leg down next to the other hip, and do this move from the other side. This time, put your thumb tips on the lower ribs, and your middle fingers on the respective iliac crests (hipbones) on the front of your neck. Now, when you lift your leg and shift it to the side, with your hands, you will be able to feel more clearly how much movement you allow in your pelvis.

The greater the movement you are undergoing, the greater the lack of abdominal recovery you are making. Even seasoned yoga students are frequently surprised by the little use they make of their abdominals in basic movements. This exercise is not only a good way to become aware of your habit of not stabilizing your abdominals while moving your legs, but it can also be a reinforcing exercise you can incorporate into your daily practice of asanas.

LIFTING ONE LEG, OUT TO THE SIDE

EXERCISE

Pelvis on a Bolster, One Leg Extended

TO CHALLENGE AWARENESS

CAUTIONS: Work bent knees to protect the lower back and to focus on the abdominals. You will feel some tightness in your abdomen that can interfere with your abdominal movement if your back doesn't bother you and you want to hold your legs straight. Do not do this exercise if you are menstruating or pregnant, or have a hiatal hernia or any strain in your eyes.

PROPS: 1 nonskid mat

If the previous exercise has been mastered you should push yourself even further. Place a padlock on your mat. Sit over the bolster on your back so that your pelvis is well protected by the bolster; your shoulders touch the floor gently; your arms are on your sides, and your knees are bent, the feet parallel and the soles on the floor.

PELVIS ON A BOLSTER, ONE LEG EXTENDED

Now, lift one leg with an exhalation and straighten it so your knees are on the same level. Without raising your pelvis, just as you did while sitting on the floor, gently shift your leg out to the side about 10 inches apart. Once again, your leg will externally rotate: that is fine. Keep your breath fast. After doing this four or five times while keeping the pelvis tight, slowly lower your leg; repeat on the other side. Notice how much more difficult it is to align your pelvis as the backbend slightly stretches out the abdominal muscles. Know that when you are in mild flexion the abdominals function best, as one of their main functions is to bring the rib cage and pelvis closer together.

YOGA ANATOMY ON HIP

The hips as a single entity include the pelvic bones, thigh bones and lowest part of the spine, which is sandwiched between the pelvic bones. This field bears the weight of the upper body and pushes it down through the legs, much like an arched stone bridge holds weight from above. The range of motion in the hip socket is limited by the depth and width of the hip socket, the shape and angle of the thigh bone and the possible tissue stress. The most effective stance for the hips and low back is to stand erect on the backline of the body, with feet parallel and shoulders. This strengthens the spine's natural curves and helps stabilize the lower body.

The most common misalignment in hips and low back is a lack of curvature at the base of the spine. This flatness creates pressure between the vertebrae on the nerves, which decreases the motion range. This flatness is also associated with the thigh bones' inward movement and the weighting of the feet's outer edges which, in turn, flakes the lower back, even more. By contrast, too much inward curvature, and not enough spine elongation, may also cause pain due to pressure on the nerves between the vertebrae. A disproportionately bent low back is associated with the femur bones' inward movement and excessive weight on the inner edges of the feet, turning the knees inward.

Hip openers facilitate root chakra movement, which can alleviate back pain in the legs which is misaligned. The hips' muscles and connective tissue contract over time and reduce the range of motion, as we preferred sitting in chairs. This combined with weak abdominal muscles (again, back support from the chair doesn't encourage abdominal region involvement) causes a situation in which many adults find it hard to sit comfortably on the ground as well.

It requires a combination of reinforcement and versatility to stretch the front and back of the hips. Standing positions such as Virabhadrasana 1 and 2 and Parsvakonasana offer a simple way of opening the hips. New or very tight students may find traditional seated hip openers such as Rajakapotasana extremely hard to estimate and difficult. In the pelvic region, the bone structure (femur heads, broader trochanter length, and acetabulum shape) can also differ considerably from student to student, allowing for some great freedom of movement and other restrictions.

TEACHER TRAINING PRACTICE ON HIP JOINTS

The femur head and the hip socket form the hip joint; the fused bones meet in the hip socket, ilium, ischium and pubis. The joint between the pubic tubercle and the upper anterior iliac spine, seen from the shoulders, lies halfway between. The hip joints and the axis through the hip joints are important for the balance and motions of the whole body. "The hip joint is a nucleus on which the entire body rotates." Through the good cooperation of all the hip-moving muscles, the balance between mobility and stability is important for hips. Particular importance is the strengthening of abductor muscles and the lengthening of iliopsoas and hamstrings. The head of the femur in standing posture does not fit into the hip socket properly. This is best done at 90 ° flexion, with some abduction and external rotation. In particular, the following points are important for balancing hip muscles and for strengthening abductor's muscles:

• Remaining inline

• Make the hips narrow as if they were pressed together

• To lengthen the hip joints before bending

• Retain the pelvic posture and keep the iliac crest line horizontal when standing on one foot

• Hold the arms perpendicular to the floor and the pelvis horizontal in four-point kneeling variants of one-legs.

The following can be practised for movement accuracy:

• Supine hip flexion sitting: sitting on the back; raising one leg, taking both hands to the shin bone. If the ilium remains unchanged the movement of the hip joint is within. If the ilium moves so that the sitting bone moves away from the surface, the iliosacral joint is involved in that. If the knee moves even further so that the area of the lumbar is flatter then the lumbar spine is also involved.

• Hip extension standing: Stand on one foot, raise the other leg backwards. Track the anterior upper iliac spine on one side of the raised shoulder, and the sacrum on the other side. Move the leg back as long as the iliac spine is not strengthened-the change is in the hip joint. The movement takes place in the iliosacral joint if the iliac spine happens going forward and backwards so the sacrum doesn't go. The movement between the sacrum and the fifth lumbar vertebra, possibly deeper into the lumbar spine, especially in a hypermobile area, when the sacrum tilts forward.

Exercise: Rhythmic external and internal rotation

Objectives: To drive the hip joints through the external and internal rotation.

1. Sit on the floor with straight legs, lengths at least two feet apart from the knees; either wear a back brace or keep your hands behind the flaps. Keeping your thighs relaxed, move your legs rhythmically, oscillating into both external and internal rotation for 1–2 minutes.

2. Sit quietly for a few breaths to end.

Variations for external and internal rotation in different planes

Sitting variation

1. Stand on an upholstered dresser.

2. Bend your elbows, so that the soles of your foot come together.

3. Place your hands on your feet or knees, your elbows straight; use a short loop around your feet if you need help sitting upright, keep your hands on the belt.

4. Rhythmically oscillate the legs like wings of a butterfly for 1–2 minutes.

5. Remain relaxed in place for a few breaths.

6. Shift your feet away from the pelvis slightly; bring your knees together and straighten your legs so that the kneecaps and toes point to the ceiling;

Exercise: Circumduction of hips

Aims: *mobilizing the hip joints, coordination.*

1. Lay on your back, and comfortably hold your head.

2. Bend your hips and knees; lift and extend your knees to your shoulders, keeping your pelvis down on the floor.

3. Hold your knee right and your knee left, with your side left.

4. Circumduct both hips contrarotating rhythmically, direct the movement of the knees with your hands; let the movements be round and smooth:

a. Start left and right circumduction at the same time, change direction in between for 5–10 breaths.

b. Start circumduction of the other side after half a circle of one hand; carry on for 5–10 breaths, changing direction in between.

5. Use the left hand to cover the right knee, the left knee with the right hand and the right arm is on top.

6. Repeat 4b, hold the wrist.

7. Turn overcrossing arms, and repeat point 4b.

8. To end the rest of calm in any symmetrical position you want for a couple of breaths.

Exercise: Hip swing

Goals: Hips stabilization and mobilization, balance.

1. Stand with your left foot, on a brick or board.

2. Keep the left hip joint stable, and hold both hips in the same place.

3. Keep your trunk upright and your arms hang loose, rhythmically swing your right leg up to 5–10 breaths

4. If you need a stability boost, stand horizontally near a wall or table to hold on with your left hand; start a few independent pendulum motions, then rise steadily.

5. Stand with your right foot on the brick or book; repeat points 2–4 on left leg.

6. Rising yourself from the pelvic floor and lower abdomen to finish standing for a few breaths with both feet on the floor.

ASANAS FOR COMMON RESPIRATORY DISORDER

To live is to breathe. Life is entirely dependent upon the breath; all living creatures, including plants, must have the air to live. 'Life is only a series of breaths' a Hindu proverb says. Breath is ever-present, from the moment a baby fills her lungs to the last breath of a dying man. Pranayama is a vital science part of yoga and its therapeutics. Pranayama is the method of breathing or controlling the motion of inhalation, exhalation and retention of vital energy.

The 'Prana' is the underlying force impregnating the whole cosmos. It is the bio-energy that activates the human body in all things; the life that makes it expand inside the seed. It's closely correlated with the air we breathe, which is our primary source of prana. But in the process of prana extraction, the air is just the physical medium to be used and managed. 'Yama' means 'power,' and pranayama is the group of techniques aimed at stimulating or controlling the vital energy. They purify the pranic body and remove blocks which allow energy to flow freely.

Pranayama provides significant advantages over the mere mechanical effect of lung exercise. It teaches us to use every part of our lungs, it strengthens our lung tissue, it relaxes our chest muscles and it energizes the system. Even Pranayama works with meditation to bring us peace and harmony with a soothing effect. The life force or Prana is referred to as the 'prana Shakthi' or 'kundalini' as a latent energy power. It exists inside the 'mooladhara' chakra. According to yoga, this prana flows from the mooladhara chakra up the spinal column to the 'Ajna chakra' between the legs.

The prana is also conveyed to the entire body through a separate set of nerve channels so it hits everybody's atom. Inhalation (puraka) strengthens the body during pranayama and fills the lungs with fresh air; retention (kumbhaka) raises the internal temperature and plays a significant role in enhancing the absorption of oxygen; exhalation (rechaka) enables the diaphragm to return to its original location, and the air full of toxins and impurities is forced out by contraction of intercostal muscles. Performance for Pranayama depends on maintaining the right inhalation, exhalation, and retention ratios.

Owing to the thick layer of immobile smoke hanging over towns caused by factories etc. the widely felt deficiency is responsible for air polluted by gas fumes and lack of sunlight. The temperature and climate that affects our body at the end of and season of the year make it normal for the person to feel exhausted. We feel particularly exhausted and worn because of the build-up of pollutants created by any physical or intellectual effort made when the atmospheric pressure is very low or when there are sudden changes in temperature; we seem to lose air and vital energy diminishes especially when the weather is sultry. Pranayama practice can counter this general build-up of toxins which paralyzes the muscles and nerves. First, pranayama cleans the body completely of toxins and then recharges it with soothing oxygen that enhances circulation.

HOW TO BREATHE PROPERLY

While we can live without food for many days, and without drinking for several hours, how many minutes will we survive without breathing? Man doesn't just have to breathe to live; he can do so in a way that keeps his health stable and avoids disease. Unfortunately, very few people know how to respire properly. As can be seen from close necks, shouldering shoulders, most people breathe in a very haphazard fashion. It was noted that unsatisfactory breathing habits would lead to respiratory disease, decreased resistance and a shorter lifespan.

Jnana mudra

This position of the finger is practised in the Pranayama exercises. In this 1mudra the index fingers are bent and folded so that either they hit the top of their respective thumbs' ends. For this article, a couple of Pranayama exercises were selected. Such exercises are easy to do, just take a couple of minutes. All should do this every day to prevent respiratory diseases. Inhale in one long, continuous movement by expanding the abdomen first, then the throat, until the full amount of air is drawn into the lungs. Then exhale, and let the lungs passively exit the air. A sense of relaxation and letting go should follow on from this. All movement from the abdomen to the chest, like a breeze, should be smooth (no jerks). This process is repeated in both inhalations and exhalations for the whole day.

NADI SHODHANA PRANAYAMA (Alternate Nostril Breathing)

How To Do?

In any comfy spot, sit comfortably. Just sit upright. Close your eyes, and remain silent. The left hand is at Jnana Mudra. Attach thumb right to the nostril. Now inhale slowly through the left nostril for a count of 5, and fill your lungs. After total inhalation, close both nostrils and hold the air in the lungs for another 5 counts. Then open the left nostril with a ring finger of the same hand, and close the left nostril. Slowly exhale to a count of 5. Open the right nostril; repeat the procedure for the same counts by closing the right nostril with the right thumb after complete exhalation through slow inhalation through the right nostril, retention and exhalation through the left nostril. One round of this loop is Nadi Shodhana Pranayama. Train 5 laps a day. Check that no sound passes through the nostrils as the air passes through them.

What good can this do?

1. Cleans the whole nervous system and tones it up.

2. People who suffer from cough and cold greatly benefit.

3. Heart fortified.

4. It cleanses irritated nostrils.

5. Removes stress and emotional stress.

6. It induces a peaceful feeling.

kapalbhati (Forceful Exhalation)

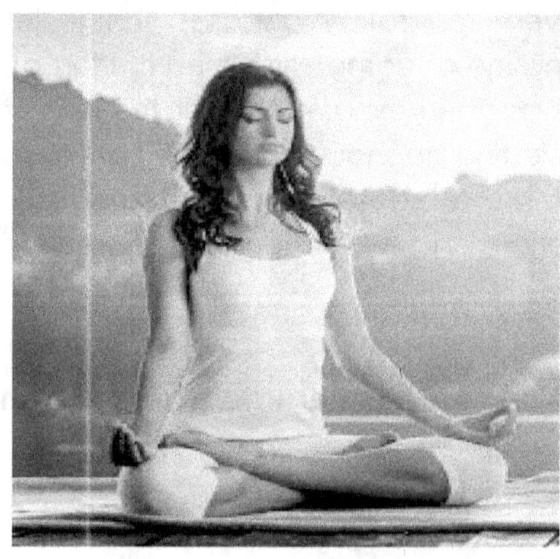

How To do?

Sit comfortably in jnana mudra, in any comfortable posture with your fingers. Chair line. Inhale both nostrils and allow contracting of the middle and lower portions of the abdomen. Rapidly expel the contractions, and then proceed with another inhalation. Simplicity and passivity breathe air. Growing frequency slowly The round takes a deep breath and steadily exhales. What could this do for good?

1. Cleans capillaries from the remotest body part.

2. Purifies the brain frontal part.

3. Aids to fight asthma, diabetes, and chronic bronchitis in addition to other nerve disorders.

4. Purifies nasal passages.

This pranayama exercise is found to be very successful as a treatment for respiratory illness. Those with pulmonary or heart issues can do this exercise only under the guidance of qualified yoga instructors.

BHRAMARI (Humming Bee Breath)

How To Do?

Sit comfortably in any comfortable position. Chair line. Inhale steadily, and deeply through the nose. By inhalation let the caress the throat area. Then place the respective index fingers gently inside the ears and close the eyes. Slowly exhale, producing a long, steady humming rhythm. Experience the sound and the sensations that were produced while breathing. This one is round. Start with 5 rounds, and gradually increase the number.

What good can this do?

1. For musicians, artists, it encourages a clear voice and is recommended.

2. Clears bacteria in the throat and nasal passage.

3. Has an impact on the mind, which creates peace and happiness.

The main purpose of Yoga is to find peace inside life. By integrating yoga into our lives, we begin with self-knowledge in our present condition and come to know the potentials and possibilities within us, and then use those strengths to attain a higher awareness in life. Pranayama, a part of Yoga, is one of the best remedies for treating respiratory diseases caused by air pollution and other respiratory diseases which occur naturally. The impact of these exercises is best achieved if completed at the start of each day. When practised in combination with asanas and meditation, pranayama helps both the body and mind to face any situation that happens in life from moment to moment.

INTRODUCTION TO CHAKRAS, NADIS AND KOSHAS

CHAKRA

Definition of chakra

The term chakra means 'wheel' or 'loop' but a better translation in the yogic sense is 'vortex' or 'whirlpool.' The chakras are vortices of pranic energy in specific areas of the body which regulate the circulation of pranas permeating the entire human structure. Can chakra is a switch that opens or activates unique areas of the brain. Such psychic centres, in most people, are latent and inactive. Concentration on the chakras enhances and helps to activate the release of energy into the chakra while performing yogic practices. This in effect awakens the dormant regions of the brain and the corresponding capacities of the spiritual and mental bodies, allowing one to achieve higher, normally inaccessible levels of consciousness.

The major chakras are numbered seven and are located along the Sushumna pathway through the centre of the spinal cord. Sushumna comes from the perineum and ends up on the head. The chakras are linked to a network of nadis called psychic channels which are more subtle but correspond to the nerves. The chakras are depicted symbolically as lotus flowers, each having a different number of petals and a characteristic colour. The lotus symbolizes the three phases of spiritual life through which the aspirant passes: ignorance, desire and enlightenment. It stands for the spiritual development from the lowest consciousness state to the highest consciousness state.

Description of the seven chakras

Mooladhara chakra: The lowest chakra is located in the perineum in the male body and the cervix in the female body. The mool word means 'heart' and adhara means 'place' And it's known as the heart hub. The chakra Mooladhara is associated with the sense of smell. It is symbolized by a deep red lotus, with four petals. In the centre are a yellow rectangle, the oiprithvi tattwa yantra, the earth element and the beeja mantra lam. In the centre of the square is a red triangle, the symbol of shakti or creative energy, with its apex pointing downwards. Within the triangle is the smoky coloured swayambhu linga which symbolizes the astral body. A red serpent representing the dormant kundalini is coiled three and a half times around the linga. The red triangle is supported by an elephant with seven trunks which symbolize the peace and unity of the earth.

Swadhisthana chakra: The swadhisthana chakra is approximately the width of two fingers in the neck above the mooladhara chakra, directly under the genital organs. The phrase's literal sense of swadhisthana is 'one's abode.' The Sanskrit word swa means 'self and that means 'place of residence.' This chakra symbolizes a six-petalled crimson lotus. In the middle are a white crescent moon, the apas tattwa yantra, the dimension of water and the beeja mantra vam. The crescent moon yantra and beeja mantra sit on a crocodile which symbolizes the subterranean movement of karmas.

Manipura chakra: Manipura chakra is found under the navel in the spine. The word mani means 'gem' and pura means 'city,' thus Manipura means 'place of jewels.' It is so-called because it is lustrous as a diamond and vibrant with vitality and power, being the centre of the fire. This chakra is depicted as a yellow lotus with ten petalled light. There is a fiery red triangle within the lotus, the tattwa yantra ol'agni, the dimension of fire and the mantra ram beeja. The ram, the emblem of energy and assertiveness, is the animal that serves as the medium for Manipura.

Anahata chakra: The Anahata chakra is situated in the spine, parallel to the nucleus, behind the sternum. The word Anahata means 'unstuck.' Sound is produced in the embodied world by striking two artefacts together, producing vibrations or sound waves. But that sound that emanates from outside this material world, the primordial sound, is the source of all sound and is known as anahadnada spiritual sound. There, in the heart centre, this sound emerges. The yogi may perceive it as the pulse of the universe, an internal, unborn, and undying vibration.

Ajna chakra: Ajna chakra is found at the top of the spine, behind the eyebrow centre, in the midbrain. Sometimes known by various names such as the third eye; jnana chakshu, the eye of wisdom; Triveni, the confluence of three rivers; guru chakra, and head of Shiva. The term Ajna stands for order. Via this chakra, the disciple receives guidance and suggestions from the guru and the divine or higher self in deeper stages of meditation.

Bindu visarga: At the top is a point known as Bindu, the back portion of the head, where a small tuft of hair grows in the Hindu brahmins. The word Bindu means 'step' or 'drop' and visarga means 'drop by drop to pour.' The spiritual centre also called soma chakra. Soma is the nectar of the gods, which is also another name of the moon. Bindu visarga is symbolized by a tiny crescent moon during a night. It is also about the production of semen.

Sahasrara: The Sahasrara lies at the head's crown. Not just a chakra, it's the abode of the highest-consciousness. The term Sahasrara means 'one thousand.' Sahasrara is visualized as a thousand-petalled sparkling lotus, containing twenty times the fifty-two Beeja mantras of the Sanskrit alphabet. In the middle of the lotus is a sparkling jyotirlinga, lingam of light, a symbol of pure consciousness. It is in Sahasrara that the divine union of Shiva and Shakti occurs, the fusion of consciousness with matter and energy, the soul of man with the supreme mind.

As kundalini awakens it ascends through the chakras to Sahasrara and fuses into the source it originates from. Matter and energy combine into pure consciousness in a state of intoxicating bliss, the purpose of yoga. Having achieved this the yogi acquires supreme knowledge, going beyond life and death.

Nadis

The word nadi means 'flow' or 'current' The ancient texts note that the mental body comprises 72 000 nadis. These are evident to a person who has developed spiritual vision as streams of light. In recent times the word nadi has been translated as 'nerve,' but nadis are composed of astral matter. Like the chakras, though referring to the nerves, they are not, in fact, part of the physical body. The Nadis are the secret channels from which the pranic forces flow. Ten are big in the psychic body out of the large number of nadis and three of these are the most significant. These are the ida, the Pingala and the Sushumna. Of these three the Sushumna is the most important. All the nadis in the mental body are Sushumna, subordially like ida and Pingala.

Ida, sushumna and pingala

Sushumna nadi, in the centre of the spinal cord, is the spiritual canal. It originates from the chakra of perineum mooladhara, and ends at Sahasrara, at the crown of the head. Ida nadi emanates from the left side of mooladhara and spirals up the spinal cord, in effect going through each chakra, forming a path of criss-cross that ends at the left side of Ajna chakra. Pingala nadi emanates from mooladhara's right side and passes in the opposite direction to that of ida, stopping at Ajna's right. The two opposing forces that exist within us are Ida and Pingala. Ida is passive, introvert and feminine; it is also known as Chandra or moon nadi. Pingala, on the other hand, is hostile, extrovert, and masculine and is called Surya, or sun nadi.

FIVE SHEATHS

1. Annamaya Kosha (Food Sheath):- It is constructed within the gross human body of elements of the physical universe. After death, it can re-enter the food cycle, produced from plants. Life, pregnancy, creation, transition, decline and death are her qualifications. Cleansing Asanas, and a balanced diet.

2. Pranamaya Kosha (Essential Sheath):- In the astral body there are five vital energies: Prana, Apana, Samana, Udana, Vyana, plus the five organs of action (karma indriyas): head, neck, feet, anus, and genitals. He faces poverty, hunger, heat and cold. Via purifying Pranayama.

3. Manomaya Kosha(Mental Sheath):-Their functions are in the astral body, mind, doubt, anger, desire, excitement, depression and illusion. Purification by the practice of yamas, nijamas and selfless devotion. It comprises of:

(A)Manas (mind)-Consideration and doubt

(B) Chitta (subconscious)-Department store

(C) eye (sight), ear (sound), nose (smell), tongue (touch), and skin (touch).

4. Vijnanamaya Kosha (Intellectual Sheath):-In the astral body, it consists of the buddhi (intellect) who analyzes and determines the true nature of every object, and the self-assertive principle of the ahamkara (ego), operating with the five

intelligence organs. It is their roles which discriminate and determine. Scriptural analysis purification, proper enquiry (Who am I?)

5. Anandamaya Kosha (Blissful Sheath):- In the causal body, he feels peace, joy, quietness and harmony. Samadhi cleaned and transcended.

TEACHER TRAINING ON TWISTING AND BINDING ASANAS

Seated and Supine Twists

Twists penetrate delightfully deep into the body's heart, stimulating and toning the internal organs, particularly the kidneys and liver, while creating softness and freedom in the spine, and opening the arms, shoulders, neck and hip. Active supine twists, such as Jathara Parivartanasana (Revolving Twist Pose), reinforce the abdominal oblique muscles which are an important group of muscles in many asanas involving rotational movements, such as Parsvakonasana (Side Angle Pose) and Astavakrasana (Eight Angle Pose).

Regular twisting helps retain the normal length and resilience of the spine's soft tissues, and the flexibility of the spine's vertebral disks and facet joints, preserving the spine's natural range of motion. In a beautiful poetic irony, we find that by turning our body into a pretzel, we can more easily unwind the accumulated physical and emotional tension trapped inside. Twists, along with this tension release, help to drive the bodymind into a more sattvic, relaxed state. Typically, however, they are neither heating nor cooling, but both: heating if it comes from a relatively cold climate, cooling if it comes from a relatively warm setting. These qualities allow us to set twists to a variety of locations in any given sequence.

Ardha Matsyendrasana (Half Lord of the Fishes Pose)

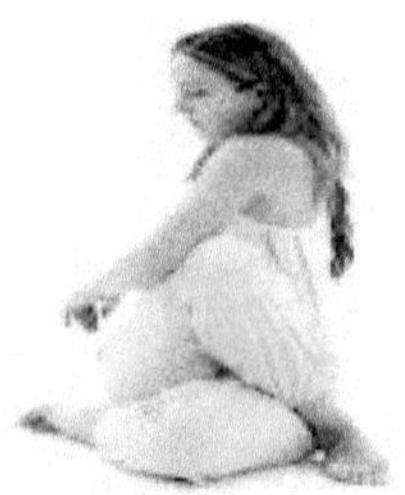

Slide the feet off Dandasana (Staff Pose) in half and bring the right heel back and down to the outside of the left leg, then put the left foot on the ground just above the right knee. Clasp both hands on the knee to lift the anterior pelvic movement and lengthen the spine by pressing down the sitting bones and left foot. Stretch the right arm to lengthen across the neck and back, then move the middle torso to the left, either clasp the left knee, extend the right elbow or back across the left knee to stabilize the twist, or stretch the right arm around the outside of the lower left leg and grip the inner left foot.

For each inhalation, step gradually out of the twist for quicker elongation of the neck, bending further with each exhale. Keep shoulder blades drawn back, heart core free, and breathe slowly. Look over to the left. Advanced students will pass through Eka Pada Koundinyasana B (One-Leg Sage Koundinya's Pose B) into the Chaturanga Dandasana (Four-Limbed Staff Pose).

Marichyasana C (Sage Marichi's Pose C)

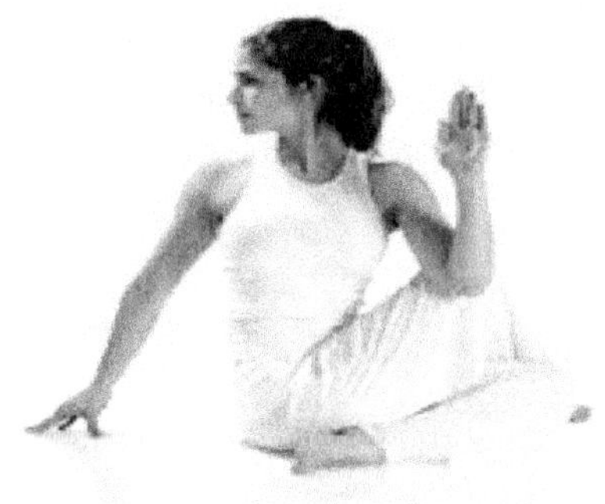

Add the right heel to the right sat bone with Dandasana 's leg lifted. Place the right hand on the floor by the right hip, reach through the spine and left shoulder and arm, then turn the body to the right, drag the left elbow of the shoulder over the right knee, causing the knee to lift the twist. For more flexibility extend the left arm around the right leg, and shine to grab the right wrist behind the back. The land stretched out across the sitting bones and the deeply engaged left thigh. For each inhalation, step gradually out of the twist for quicker elongation of the neck, bending further with each exhale. Keep shoulder blades drawn back, heart core free, and breathe slowly. Look over to the left. Advanced students will pass through Eka Pada Bakasana (One-Leg Crane Pose) into Chaturanga Dandasana.

TEACHER TRAINING PRACTICE ON SHOULDER JOINTS

The two clavicles and the scapulae form the shoulder-girdle. Glenohumeral joints, the ball and socket joints that connect the scapula and the humerus are the most flexible and least stable joints in the body. A thorough assessment should be based on finding out if the restriction is in the scapulothoracic area or if it compensates for weakness or hypermobility in the glenohumeral joint before suggesting a specific exercise routine for the shoulder girdle. In such cases, the further mobilization of the glenohumeral joint can cause discomfort, although the scapulae 's mobility is also advantageous. Strong blades in the shoulder aid in weight-bearing defence. And the clavicles are relocalized in most shoulder exercises.

Other structures related to the shoulder girdle also exist, from the skull to the pelvic. Such areas are worth considering as well, particularly if research on the shoulder girdle itself is not improving. A common cause of shoulder problems is a restriction at the upper ribs. Rib-mobilizing training is clever, then. Since the anatomical structures and functions of the cervicothoracic junction are closely connected to the shoulder girdle, here we will define these two regions.

Exercise: Pendulum exercises standing

Objectives: To strengthen the shoulder joints, in particular, to facilitate the movement of fluids.

1. Stand up in a natural position with one step apart from the knees, one foot forward, one foot backwards, the front leg bent slightly.

2. To move your pelvis as if you were walking, slightly lift your heel back and then drop it down to the floor.

3. Swing your arms at a regular speed like a pendulum up to 1 minute in opposition; be mindful of the weight of your arms.

4. Shift your feet and swing your arms, as set out in item 3.

Exercise: Scapular movements

Objectives: mobilization of the shoulder blades, relaxation of the periscapular region, coordination.

1. Sit down on the floor, cross-legged, or sit parallel to your knees and feet on a chair; change your lumbopelvic position.

2. Maintaining a well balanced neutral stance and head, move the blades of the shoulder in various directions, for 3–5 breaths each:

a. Forward (apart from each other) and reverse (closer)

b. Up And Down

c. Circular (in a horizontal and counterclockwise direction). Keep after each movement for a few breaths; feel the rhythm of breathing between your shoulder blades, and relax your shoulders.

Tips

• Switch hands in the opposite direction and practice equal balance.

• You'll be more mindful of the gesture when a friend puts his hands on your shoulder blades and watches your actions.

• It also helps to improve vision by executing wall-leaning scapular motions.

YOGA ANATOMY ON SKELETAL SYSTEM

The Skeletal System performs many important functions; it provides the structure and shapes for our bodies besides supporting, protecting, facilitating body movement, providing blood for the body and storing minerals.

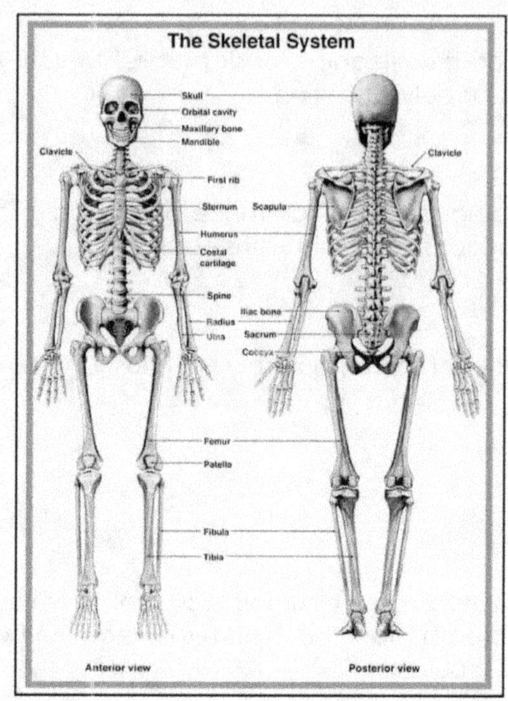

Functions

The 206 bones form a rigid structure, attached to the softer tissues and organs of the body. The Skeletal System contains vital organs. The underlying skull protects the brain while the heart and lungs are surrounded by the sternum and rib cage. The body movement is dealt with by the muscle and skeleton systems. Therefore they are often known as the network of the musculoskeletal. Muscles are joined up to the bones by tendons. Bones are tied together by ligaments. Usually, it is called a joint where bones touch. Two separate bones are attached to muscles causing joint movement and contract together to keep them together. One example will be the contraction of biceps and the relaxation of triceps. This creates a curve in the elbow.

The contraction of the triceps and relaxation of the biceps produces the effect of straightening up the arm. The marrow contained in some bones contains blood cells. The bone marrow produces an average of 2.6 million red blood cells per second to replace those that the liver stripes and destroys. Bones serve as a storage place for minerals, including calcium and phosphorous. If there is a blood deficit, accumulation may occur within the bones. If these minerals are poorly available within the blood, the supply would be replenished from the bones.

Axial Skeleton: Skull (not every single bone), vertebral cord, bony thorax (rib cage).

-- The skeleton consists of 7 cervical, 12 thoracic and 5 vertebral lumbar

-- The spine has many natural curvatures characteristic of it. The sacrum is convex to the left. The lumbar is very concave. The chestnut is convex. The area around the cervix is concave.

-- Scoliosis is a lateral vertebral curvature.

--Ribs We have seven real, three fake, two floating.

Appendicular Skeleton:

-- On the upper and lower extremities

-- Shoulder-girdle bones and limbs

-- Pelvic gill bones and legs

-- The wristbones are carpal and the bones of the foot are tarsals.

Classification of Joints

-- Synovial Joint Styles

• Joint hinge Ex:- Elbow

· Ex ball and socket:-

· Intercarpal Gliding Ex:-

· Ellipsoid Ex:- Atlas-overs

· Atlas-axis pivot Ex:

Á Saddle Ex:- Metacarpal Carpal

Composite Structure of a Typical Synovial Joint

Terms of Movements

-- Bending

-- Expand

-- Retrieval

-- Adding

-- Wheeling

-- Outside / Lateral Movement

-- Indoor / medial spin

-- Surprise

-- The Pronunciation

-- Horizontal twist

-- Horizontal distribution

-- Retirement

-- Freezing

-- Lifting

-- Flexion on dorsal

-- Flflexion in plantar

-- Tumbling

-- Lateral twist

PRACTICE ON ADVANCE ASANAS ON BALANCING POSES

No effort should be made towards the advanced level of asana unless the body is very flexible. Before attempting to perform any of these postures, asanas must be taught in the beginners and intermediate classes. It is important to avoid stressing the body while performing advanced asanas in any way. Such procedures require that the limbs and joints travel into unfamiliar positions which are not used to. Any pressure could affect them. Gently coaxing the body over some time to perform advanced asanas is much easier than punishing attempts to achieve immediate results.

UTTHAN EKA PADA SIRASANA

Utthan Eka Pada Sirasana

(standing foot to head pose)

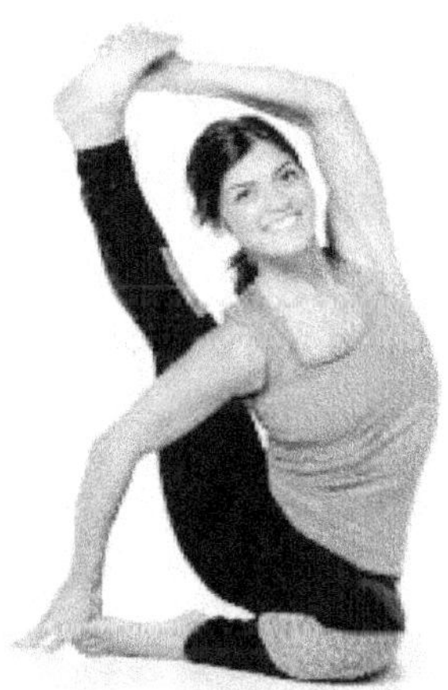

Lie down on the ground, with legs stretched out. Bend your left knee, and place your left foot outside on the left buttock. Assume Eka pada sirasana with right leg behind the back. Using the supporting hands and arms to place each of the palms on the floor. Lean back slightly and get left in a squatting position. Keep your leg straight, and get upright. Don't put on the pressure. When the balance is retained in the standing position, bring the palms above the chest together. This is the closing line. Keep balance in standing posture as long as it is convenient. Sit attentively, and lower the raised knee. Stretch the arm out, and relax. Repeat backwards, on the other hand.

Breathing: Inhale as the body uplifts. In the final place, of course, breathe. Exhale as down the neck.

Sequence: We can only attempt this asana after we have mastered Eka pada sirasana.

Consciousness: uplifting the body physically to a state of uprightness, regular breathing in the final position, and maintaining equilibrium. Anahata Spiritual Chakra-On.

Other details: As for pada eka sirasana.

Practice note: Since balancing in this pose is very difficult, you can need to ask for help from a friend or make use of a wall at the beginning.

Padma Mayurasana (lotus or bound peacock pose)

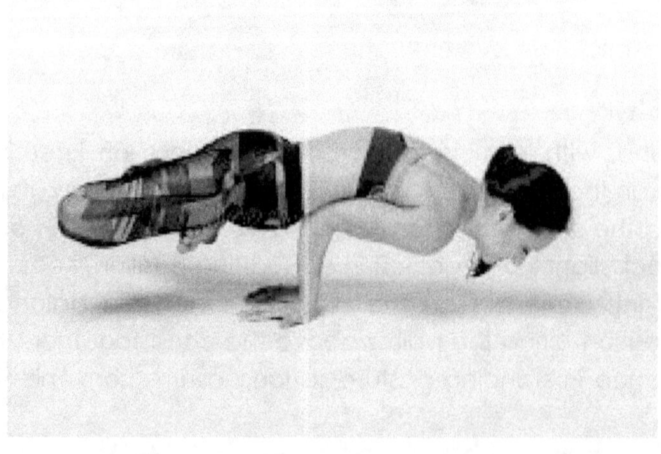

Sit down in padmasana, and mentally relax the whole body. Body development uses hands to carry the weight of the feet. Place the palms flat on the floor in front of the body, with the fingers pointing down to the knees. Bending and bringing in the elbows. Step forward, aligning the elbows on either side of the abdomen. Lean-to the upper arms higher, so that the chest rests. Find Equilibrium Point for the body. Lean in more and steadily raise the folded legs from the floor. Don't put on the pressure. The body, head, and legs should lie in a straight line, horizontal. That's the start line. Keep the place comfortable for a certain time. Gradually lower the knees, and return to starting position. Adjust the position of the legs, make the upper leg in the opposite direction and do another round.

Other details: Mayurasana in its present form.

Practice note: If the practitioner can sit in padmasana comfortably, performing Padma mayurasana is easier than the basic pose of mayurasana, particularly for females.

HANUMANASANA

Hanumanasana (Hanuman's pose)

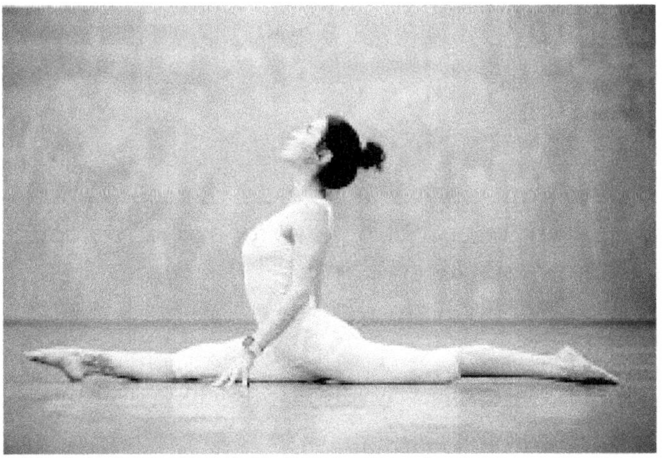

Kneel on the left knee, and position the right foot about 30 cm in front of the left knee. Place the palms of hand on the deck, on either side of the right foot. Slide slowly and gradually forwards the right foot. Carries body weight on feet at the same time. Straighten both legs and drive as far as possible the right foot forward, and the left as far back as without pain. In the final position, the buttocks are lowered so that the pelvic floor and both legs rest on the table in one straight line. Close your eyes, relax your body and bring your hands together against the sternum. Check the knee straight behind. Keep the spot safe for as long as possible. Return to Start Place. Repeat forwards asana with the other leg.

Breathing: Breath normally all day.

Duration: Once per hand.

Awareness: muscles of the physical-on leg and relaxing of air.

Spiritual mooladhara chakra-on ajna, or anahata.

Sequence: After completing this asana, sit on with both legs stretched forward for one or two minutes.

Contra-indications: It is strictly recommended that people suffering from conditions such as slipped disk, sciatica, hernia and hip joint dislocation should not attempt this asana.

Benefits: This stance makes the legs and hips more flexible, and the blood pumps. It massages the abdominal organs, tones the reproductive system and makes the female body ready for childbirth.

Practice note: The greatest measure for flexibility in legs and hips is Hanumanasana. Very few people will be able to lower the body down to the floor in final position. Those who can't place a pillow under the pelvic floor or folded blanket to prevent strain.

VISHWAMITRASANA

Vishwamitrasana (Sage Vishwamitra's pose)

Stand straight with arms secured by the sides and feet. Close your eyes, and physically relax your whole body. Open the eyes, progressively lean forward from the knees and place the palms on the floor next to the feet. With the buttocks lifted, take the legs back about 120 to 150 cm without moving the hands and position the crown of the head on the floor. Head up, cross the right leg over the right hand and bring the right thigh back on the upper right arm back. It doesn't hit the ground with the right foot. Immediately turn the body to the left, and place the left arm along the left thigh and balance.

Switch left to foot sideways and bring the heel on the board. Just straighten your knee correctly. Stretch the left arm vertically from the hip and look upward bent to the left side. This is the closing line. Keep till you feel comfortable. Relive the right leg and head back to the starting point. Repeat the pose for the same period on the other hand.

Breathing: Inhale as the neck goes upwards. Exhale, as the limb goes back.

Duration: One time at each side, holding position for up to 30 seconds.

Awareness: Putting physical on.

Spiritual mooladhara chacra-on.

Benefits: This asana extends and strengthens the muscles of the arms and legs, and the sciatic nerves. It strengthens internal organs, increases concentration and enhances balance.

YOGA ANATOMY ON THE SPINE ALIGNMENT

The central nervous system allows for an enormous amount of versatility in the survival activities of a vertebrate with its complex sensory and motor functions. As these structures developed over millions of years and became more essential to the survival of our early ancestors, they needed the necessary development of a protective structure that allows for free movement but is robust enough to protect these important but fragile tissues. The structure, the skeleton, is perhaps the most elegant and complex solution per description for the dual requirements of sthira and sukha. Of all mammals, the human spine is unique because it exhibits both primary and secondary curves.

The primary spine curve consists of the kyphotic thoracic and sacral curves; the lumbar and cervical regions have parallel, lordotic curves. Only a real biped has both sets of curves; tree-swinging and knuckle-walking primates have some curve of the cervix but no lumbar lordosis, which is why they can not move comfortably on two legs straight. The key curve (kyphotic) was the first front-back spinal curve that appeared as aquatic creatures made the transition to the sea. The entire spine is in a primary curve as a person waits in utero for its emergence from its watery roots. It changes shape for the first time when the head reaches the hairpin curve of the birth canal, and for the very first time the neck feels the secondary (lordotic) curve.

As the postural development progresses from the head downwards, the cervical curve continues to evolve until you start holding up the weight of your head at about three to four months, and when you begin to sit upright, it evolves entirely about nine months. To carry the weight over the feet, you have to grow a lumbar curve by walking and creeping on the floor for months.

At 12 to 18 months, as you begin walking, the lumbar spine straightens out of its dominant, kyphotic curve. The lumbar spine starts to become concave forward (lordotic) by the age of 3 years, but this will not be evident to the outside until age 6-8. Only after age 10 is the lumbar curve fully approaching its adult form.

TEACHERTRAINING ON LOWER-MID BACK SPINE ALIGNMENT

A thorough diagnosis is needed because a lot of different pathologies can cause low back pain. Particular caution is needed if neurological signs and symptoms are associated with the low back pain, problems with the bowel and bladder, or if the patient has lost weight or feels ill. If exercise therapy is required after a thorough medical examination, the general function of the lumbar spine must be taken into account as a weight-bearing structure that must be capable of increasing against gravity and changing direction, and well balanced. Exercises require enhancement and mobilization.

Exercise: Stability at the Lumbopelvic

Objectives: to improve lower abdomen, pelvic floor and lumbar region.

1. Lie on your back with your hips and knees bent, feet sole on the ground, heels away from the buttocks one-foot high. Wearing a pillow for your back if needed.

2. Gently turn the pelvis until it is neutral to the lumbopelvic spot. Keep the position unchanged over the following sequence of exercises.

3. Place your fingertips on the central line of your lower abdomen, about 5 fingers under your navel. Relaxing your neck and arms, pull this lower abdominal area slightly inwards when you exhale into your lumbar spine; feel the gradual contraction of the lower abdomen under your fingertips. Typically then inhale while holding the abdomen relaxed.

4. Do point 3-5 times, with 1–2 natural breaths in between if necessary. You can feel the pelvic floor movement associated with that, as well as the lumbar area.

5. Repeat with an exhalation, maintain the contraction for up to 3 seconds, and release it while exhaling.

6. Take a few breaks and relax.

7. Relax your throat and arms, practice the gentle contracting motion of point 3 as you inhale; relax as you exhale; feel the subtle contraction with your fingertips on the middle line of the lower abdomen.

8. Do 3–5 times point 7.

9. Hold the contraction again for 3 minutes, and release it with relaxed hands while exhaling.

10. For a few seconds, remain calm; feel the softness in your pelvic floor and abdomen;

Refined work

Resting your arms on the floor behind your body obey points 2–10 without fingertips guiding the lower abdomen.

ASANAS FOR NECK JOINT

We have listed together these three fields since they are closely related. The system of stomatognathy is called the head, neck, and jaw. All the muscles that bind these areas and the shoulder girdle are working together in a continuous, complex way. "The efficiency of this balancing mechanism results in effective mouth, chest, cervical spine and head function, as well as the thorax and upper limb function." The hyoid bone plays a central role in this system; it binds the shoulder, mandible and cranium girdle. In cases where there are problems with the temporomandibular joint, a first dental examination should be carried out. Also, gentle local mobilisation often reduces stress. In some cases, the posture and activity patterns of certain areas of the body are involved and need rectification. The mandibular can move up and down on both sides, back and forth. These two motions are combined at chewing. The mandible goes forth when you open your mouth; when the mouth is closed, it moves backwards.

Exercise: Atlas and axis

Objective: Mobilisation of the upper cervical spine.

1. Lie down relaxed on your back with your abdomen and lumbar region, relax your shoulders and rest your head comfortably; use a pillow for your head if necessary.

2. When you exhale, turn the head very softly to the right; bring it back to the centre with the inhalation, lengthening the face slightly.

3. Turn the head to the left very softly as you exhale; move it back with the inhalation to the centre, lengthening the face slightly.

4. Do 2 and 3, 3–5 times, then pause for a few breaths.

Exercise: Longneck

Objective: To hold the cervical spine against gravity for long.

1. Sit straight on the floor or on a chair; place a book or small bag filled with flour or rice or another suitable object on the crown of your head.

2. Feel as you inhale the rising and lengthening as if you lift the object higher on your head; hold this lifting up during exhalation.

3. Holding the pelvis neutral and relaxing the shoulders, continuously finetune the head location so the weight on the crown of the head remains secure.

4. If it feels good, hold this lift for 3–5 breaths, or longer.

Exercise: Strong neck

Aim: general cervical spinal strengthening.

1. Sit on the floor upright, or in a chair.

2. Place one hand on your forehead so you can't turn your head forward.

3. Apply no more than 10–30 per cent of your maximum strength so you can keep your usual breathing; retain the resisted position for 2–3 breaths; remove your hand and relax your arms for 2–3 breaths, lengthening your cervical spine.

4. Do points 2 and 3 2–3 times; repeat with the opposite hand.

5. Place both hands with the fingers interlocked on the back of your head to stop back-bending of your head.

6. Apply no more than 10–30 per cent of your full strength to keep your normal breathing; hold the resisted position for 2–3 breaths; drop your hands and relax your arms for 2–3 breaths, lengthening your cervical spine.

7. 2–3 Put points 5 and 6 into effect.

8. Bring your left hand over your mouth, and put it over your right ear.

9. Do not bend your head sideways to the right with no more than 10–30 per cent of your maximum power, so you can continue your regular breathing; keep your resisted position for 2–3 breaths; release your hand and relax your arms for 2–3 breaths, lengthening your cervical spine.

10. 2–3 Execute points 8 and 9.

11. For the other side repeat points 8–10.

12. Place your right hand on your forehead and your left hand on the back of your head; this way, the palms avoid the movement of your head to the right.

13. Keep for 2–3 seconds, then get your hands off.

14. Make points 12 and 13 2–3 times.

15. Shift your hands and execute points in the other direction 12–14.

16. Keep sitting to finish and relax for a few breaths.

TEACHING METHODOLOGY FOR HAMSTRING AND KNEE JOINTS

Perhaps the hardest joint to the body is the knee. It is the largest joint of the synovial joints, such joints containing a lubricant fluid enclosed in a capsule. The knee must also deal with the weight-bearing from above and the force-absorption from below, as does the shoulder. The menisci increase the surface area for these functions, thus increasing stability. Ligaments and muscles are essential to stability. The exercises will not only enhance muscle strength but will also enhance coordination and healthy cooperation among the different muscle groups. For it is vital to align the kneecaps and feet, knee joints and ankle joints through exercise: good function is equally required.

The full range of movement is important for the cartilage and menisci to get the best nutrition. We have talked about the stability before. The main moves are flexion and extension: the secondary moves are limited ranges of internal and external rotation, abduction, and adduction. There's also a minor function to translation. A slight rotation of the outer tibia increases knee flexibility when extending the knee. One can see and feel a slight outward movement of the tibial tuberosity, or the lower leg can be held steady and the thigh turned slightly inward. The extended knee is locked to full by both movements. Activities are conceived to improve both stability and motion. The results are achieved not only through the acts themselves but also through the consistency of the gestures, which should be smooth.

Finetuning, loosening slightly from the limit of motion, helps to stay within the functional range and to use the muscles in a controlled, organized way. This means a limited flexion combined with an extension to the knee which is fully extended. You can add a minimum stretching action, such as resisting the bending motion, when bending the knees. Such acts particularly apply to stand up. In short, the muscles of the flexor and the extensor are a controlled operation.

Exercise: Knee movement with rhythm

Aims: mobilizing the knee joints, facilitating fluid mobility.

1. Sit just on a bed.

2. The lower legs oscillate rhythmically forward and reverse for 1–3 minutes.

3. Relax on lower legs for a few breaths.

4. Rhythmically circumduce the lower legs for 1–3 minutes, so that the legs can swing; adjust the direction in between.

5. Relax upon the lower legs for a few breaths.

Exercise: Knee extension fine-tuning

Aims: Complete knee joint extension, flexor balance and muscle extensor control.

1. Sit on concrete, feet in dorsiflexion, with straight legs.

2. When you need it, use a back brace, or place your hands on the floor behind your pelvis.

3. Hyperextend the two knees, alternating with a bending trace 3–5 tImes.

4. Keep the knee extension contact with a bending trace for 3–5 breaths, hold the foot in dorsiflexion, and spread the toes out.

5. Relax arms and legs; stay on for a few breaths.

Exercise: Mobile patella

Aims: *mobilizing the kneecaps, coordination.*

1. Sit on the floor with straight legs and feet dorsiflex; use a backrest if necessary; place your fingertips around the kneecaps to feel the motion.

2. Continue breathing naturally, contract rhythmically and relax your thigh muscles to move your kneecaps, 5–10 times, contract both sides simultaneously, then repeat 5–10 times between left and right.

3. Contract the muscles in the thigh; maintain the contraction to 3–5 breaths; add a hint of knee joint flexion.

4. Gradually the thighs let go; let them relax for 1–2 breaths.

5. 3 and 4 happen 3-5 times.

Variation

Perform 2–5 points while standing.

Exercise: Posterior knee

Aims: *mobilizing the knee joints, relaxing the back of the knee.*

1. Use a pelvis brace that is high enough to raise the right leg to sit down on the floor, with the toes pointing upward with both buttocks leaning on the brace equally; the left toes pointing to the ceiling.

2. Lift your right buttock slightly so that the right palm and flat fingers can be put on the calf; the fingers contact the back of the knee.

3. When you lower your right buttock, pull the calf muscle away from the back of the knee and sideways very gently with your fingertips; then withdraw your right hand from the calf.

4. Rest equal on both sides.

5. Place the right palm on the right thigh and the left palm on the left thigh; 3–5 breaths remain.

6. Place the sole on the right foot floor with the knee pointing to the ceiling and move away from the right heel to extend the hip, keeping the knee soft.

7. Repeat points 1–6 on the left leg.

8. To end the sitting with both legs straight for a few breaths, with the kneecaps and toes pointing to the ceiling.

Exercise: Rotation of the lower leg

Aims: *mobilizing the knee joint into the rotation and stabilizing it.*

1. Sit on a chair with more than hip-width apart from the knees and feet, and perpendicular to the floor shin bones.

2. Put your left hand on your right thigh above your knee; hold your fingers on the outside of your forearm; your right hand is around the top of your right shin bone.

3. Turn your right foot inward and outward, 5–10 times, using your right pivoting heel.

4. Your left side stabilises the right thigh.

5. On the tuberosity of the shin bone, you can sense the rotational motion of the lower leg with your right side.

6. Start stabilizing right thigh with your left hand.

7. Repeat right foot motion as set out in point 3, with rotation resistant to the right hand.

8. For left knee, repeat 2–7 points.

9. Keeping your knees and feet parallel, slightly apart, aligned correctly to complete the sitting straight for a few minutes.

Exercise: Stable knees

Aims: *stabilizing the knee joints, connecting with pelvic stability.*

1. Lie comfortably balanced with your head on your back, your legs straight and your feet comfortable.

2. Tilt your pelvis so that the lumbar spine gets closer to the ground; you can feel that movement with your hands on your front hip bones.

3. Also, tilt your pelvis and start bending your knees.

4. Keep the pelvic position; stretch the legs at a time.

5. Rest for 1–2 breaths.

6. Release the pelvis' backwards tilt slightly only to the point where it feels relaxed in the lumbar region and back of the pelvis; relax the legs and feet.

7. Do 2–6 3–5 points.

8. In dorsiflexion, repeat points 2–7, with your feet.

9. Keep relaxed on the concrete for a few minutes, feeling the back touch of your pelvis and the back of your legs.

ETHICS OF YOGA TEACHER, MORALITY AND DISCIPLINE

The Yamas and Niyamas of the classical Ashtanga Yoga method offer concise, and yet very true instructions to students.

Niyamas and Yamas

Yamas (Ethical Disciplines): These ethical principles include our relationship with others, our external environment and existence.

Ahimsa (Non-harmful): kindness to others; compassion; non-obstruction of the flow of nature; gentleness and non-violence to others and ourselves.

Satya (Truthfulness): being true to ourselves; being fair and upright; denying the truth, or playing or exaggerating.

Asteya (Non-stealing): don't take what isn't yours; don't hoard; don't give your full because of someone else.

Bramacharya (Walking or having ethical conduct like God): to relate to others with complete integrity and lack of manipulation; to be conscious of sexual desires and to properly channel that energy.

Aparigraha (Non-clinging): have an open hand and an open heart; live on our property easily and without any unwanted connection.

Niyamas (Internal Restrictions) — These are ethical rules that include daily practices, behaviour, attitude and communication.

Saucha (Purity): cleanliness, honesty, optimistic disposition and equanimity of mind.

Santosha (Contentment): recognition of circumstances; peace with one another and with oneself.

117

Tapas (heat): self-discipline for a deeper relationship with our divinity; a purifying fire within.

Svadhyaya (Self-examination): the search for divinity by careful self-analysis and scriptural study; an open-minded investigation of the world's nature and ourselves as its microcosm.

Ishvara Pranidhana: submission to the higher power of consciousness and willingness to serve.

More on the Ethics of a Teacher

We as teachers hold an honorary role and thus have a responsibility for our students. With modesty, we are giving our voice as part of a tradition of our teachers. Every teacher too is a pupil. As teachers, we aim to promote and create barriers as well to direct the student's energies. Anything that we do that detracts from the student's ability to focus on yoga art should not be a part of our teaching. Developing a bond with the students is normal, honourable and to be expected. There is an imbalance of power within the relationship between student and teacher. If there is love between a teacher and a student, these feelings should not be acted upon automatically. Perhaps the best option to try is to find another competent teacher for a student with whom you may think a relationship might develop.

TEACHING METHODOLOGY FOR SPECIAL PEOPLE

Yoga is one of six oldest schools of Indian philosophy. It's the practice that enables one to achieve higher levels of success, bringing out the latent potentials from within. Yoga's daily practice will enhance both physiological and psychological well-being. Disability changes the way people are treated towards the mind. They have a poor self-image and lack faith. They grow emotions of inferiority from their understanding of their failure and lack of performance in all ways. They are frustrated because they are unable to perform simple tasks, either not at all or with considerable difficulty.

So they're still very nervous and tired of physical exertion. The spine is rigid and thus causes a lot of pain and also limits mobility, imbalances in coordination. They have issues with the publicity, too. This is better done on a one-to-one basis while using Yoga as a Therapy. A human study of yoga therapy is limited in children with different disabilities. Further studies are required to confirm those results. Surya Namaskar can provide simple Jathis and Kriyas as part of the warm-up practices. This helps to improve flexibility in the body.

ASANAS: Although children may not be able to do all poses 'differently' and there are some positions which are of particular benefit to them. Even trying to attain a specific pose has the same advantage as getting to the final position. Depending on the type of impairment, each of those postures may be modified for them. They can be taught doing various poses without moving at all. There are examples of chronically disabled people who perform their yoga exercise using their beds or wheelchairs. Asanas work on the muscles and joints, creating space within the body's structure to help improve mobility and flexibility. There are less tension and more organized physical activity.

Postures to boost blood flow to the head: Postures such as Viparitkarani, Sarvangasana, Matsyasana, Halasana and Suptavajrasana alternating with standing positions such as Padahastasana, Trikonasana, Padangushtasana help to increase blood flow to the head area and can help activate the brain cells.

Concentration-increasing postures: postures such as Vrikshasana, Natarajasana and Ardhachakrasana are balanced. To maintain these postures, the parent or the teacher must support the children.

Postures to improve trust and body position: Back bending postures such as Bhujangasana, Ushtrasana, Chakrasana, Dhanurasana which opens up the shoulders and region of the chest are useful for improving their body position and self-confidence. To those affected by the weakness of the lower extremities may be taught the practice of hand-balancing postures. These children are especially good at those poses. Simhasana improves the stammering, stuttering and some defects in the tongue, nose, and throat of infants. Pavanamukta Asana is also a pleasurable practice.

Thus, beginning from simple movements and dynamic postures, they can be slowly carried on to the static postures, the Sthira and Sukha concept, and thus slowly fulfilled. The explanation is more successful than just explaining. (This holds all the good Yogic Techniques). Postures are adjusted according to the strengths of each boy.

PRANAYAMA: Pranayama directs and controls breathing, and greatly benefits people with disabilities. This technique especially enhances stamina, flexibility and strength along with enhanced Vital Energy circulation promoting better sleep. Healthy breathing can also help to alleviate deep emotional and physical tension within the body. Pranayama helps to handle fits which may be popular among these children. Animal sounds make their performance interesting. A favourite of all time is Kukkuriya Pranyama, (dog panting breath) with girls. Mathangi Pranayama, with Cheeri and Sharabha Kriya in Vyagraha Pranayama. Even other people like Kapalabhati are very useful (for the slow, not the hyperactive). The Shitali and Sitkari Pranayama are helpful to the people affected by the Down's syndrome because with speech impairment they have thickened the tongue. Mukha Bhastrika is also known as the 'cleansing breath' which helps remove old polluted air from the lungs and cleans the bloodstream of excess carbon dioxide. His practice also decreases reaction time and improves memory and comprehension.

SHATKARMAS: Some of the Shatkarmas such as Trataka, Kapalabhati, may be very useful for concentration development and may even act as tranquillisers. These children suffer from numerous eye-related issues, and Trataka and the Neti, along with a diet rich in vitamin A and C, are extremely beneficial for these children.

MUDRAS: Bhujangini Mudra and Brahma Mudra, working with breath and sound vibration creates a sense of relaxation and reinvigorates the area of the head and neck reducing tension, Hasta Mudras and Kaya Mudras(Yoga Mudra, Manduka Mudra) help push away depression, bringing forth a sense of happiness and joy. Stop Oli Mudras due to its strong effects on gonadal and other endocrine glands.

BANDHA: de Jalandhara bandha. Might include Uddiyana Bandha later on.

DHYANA: Practicing any form of meditation reduces feelings of isolation and gives peace of mind. It is also ideal for the disabled physically but a psychologically demanding activity.

YOGIC RELAXATION: Homeland and abroad, unreasonable expectations bring a strong social pressure to drive them insane. With Kaya Kriya and Spanda-Nishpanda Shava Asana relaxes all aspects of the musculoskeletal system. Simple mantras of prayer and chanting make them less violent, purify speech, relax the mind and help minimize stress. These children will benefit from chanting the Pranava Mantra AUM. Helps with rest to maintain their focus and increase their alertness, and enables them to develop mental and emotional energy.

BENEFITS OF THE YOGA PRACTICES

Living Yoga is important to understand and make it a way of life. Yoga helps them to coordinate the activities of mind, body and emotions, reduces the disturbed state of mind by helping them to focus and concentrate, improves the activities of today's life to the degree that could never otherwise be accomplished, improves their ability and helps them to rely on themselves to make them independent, helps them to develop their social relations, reduces their ability.

TEACHING METHODOLOGY ON PELVIC MUSCLES

The pelvis consists of two innominated bones, each fused with three bones: ilium, ischium, and pubis. The pelvis covers the pelvic and abdominal organs along with a complex soft tissue system; in women, the pelvis also helps carry and give birth to a baby. The pelvis must absorb dynamic, asymmetric forces from below and forces carrying weight from above. The pelvis joints are the symphysis pubis and the sacroiliac or iliosacral joints depending on which bone we find to be stable and which is moving. No other area of the body could have been debated just as much as the sacrum and its ilia joints. There are innumerable varieties of sacrum shapes, and movement and joint planes. Mobility decreases with age, presumably because of increased calcification of the ligaments. There is generally less versatility in men than there is in women.

Ligamentous stability also affects female hormonal changes. You may passively and actively move both the innominate bones and the sacrum. For active movements muscles are attached to the innominates and the sacrum. Even the sacrum can behave in many different ways. The anteroposterior angle of the sacrum is connected to curves within the spinal cord. Vertebral columns with more prominent curves on a near-vertical sacrum are often more mobile than less curved columns but both can perform well.

Exercise: Correcting pelvic torsion

Aim: *derotating the pelvis.*

To check the side of the pelvic is more rear or left, on which side it is rotated:

1. Sit on the sidelines.

2. Bend both knees, keep your feet on the concrete sole, and all knees and feet together.

3. Rock both knees at a slow rhythm towards the left and right.

4. If you have more weight in your right hip while you rock to the right than in your left hip when you rock to the left, your right side is more reverse; so your left side is more forward.

Here we explain the exercise for a rear right side; if your left side is more central, in the definition, swop left and right:

1. Lie down comfortably on the floor, using a pillow to your back if you need it.

2. Bend your right leg, knee towards your chest; grip both hands on the back of your thigh or the top of your shin; hold your thigh back if there is any knee pain.

3. Keep your shoulders relaxed on the floor, bring your right leg up to your body.

4. Lift your left leg, move it outwards around your foot's width to the left and slowly lower it to the floor; the left leg's weight flips your pelvis to the left – as opposed to the reported pelvic rotation.

5. Return your left leg to starting position along the left side of your body.

6. Push your right leg much more into your chest, and repeat points 4 and 5.

7. Repeat study mentioned above.

8. If improvement happens repeat points 2–7 once or twice, depending on the outcome.

9. After the test is over, relax in a symmetrical position for a few breaths.

Exercise: Mobilization of the iliosacral joints

Aims: *mobilizing the iliosacral joints, moving the ilium posteriorly.*

1. Lying on your back; if you need it, use an acceptable pillow under your ear.

2. Hold your left leg straight, lift your right knee to the right side of your chest, so that the hip falls off the ground; bring both hands to your neck back.

3. Keep on for 2–3 breaths, then slowly release, hold your hands in place and stay there for 1–2 breaths.

4. Sit down on the floor with your right arm; keep your left shoulder relaxed; put your left hand around the back of your right thigh close to your knee or the top of your shine; put your right knee closer to your stomach, slightly to your left side;

5. Hold on for 2–3 breaths, then slightly release, retain right-hand spot, and stay there for 1–2 breaths.

6. Bring your right knee closer to your stomach, adducting more to your left shoulder; the right hip comes further away from the floor.

7. Hold on for 2–3 seconds, then release your hands and return to asymmetric posture, either with your legs bent or straight, whichever you feel more comfortable; feel if there is any difference in how the left and right hips are on the floor.

8. Repeat points 2–7 on the left leg.

YOGIC STUDY ON MUSCULAR SYSTEM

Muscle governs virtually all body movements. It moves bones at the joint muscles. The two surfaces of the bone to which it is connected get closer together (by a tendon) as a skeletal muscle contract or shorten. Muscle cells are a tightly structured system that the connective tissue called fascia keeps together and divides. This fascia allows for the effortless passage of muscle fibres and is continuous throughout the body. Inside the muscle cell, there are striated bundles which can be compared to small train box cars on tracks called filaments. When a contraction occurs the boxcars get closer together (myosin filament = rail tracks; actin filament = box cars).

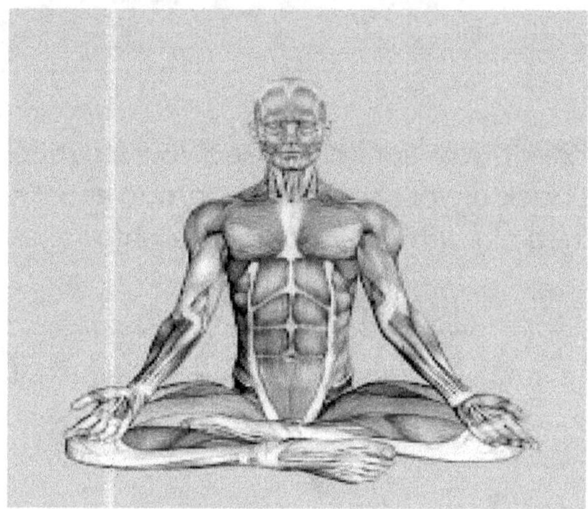

Pull muscles; never push. Because of this linear structure, one can deduce the direction of motion by viewing the connection sights of the muscle-tendon. As the muscle contracts, the distance between those two points will decrease. This is largely due to the balance of complimentarily opposing muscles working together in the union when a joint is in perfect alignment, where there is enough space, minimal tension and cohesion with the rest of the body.

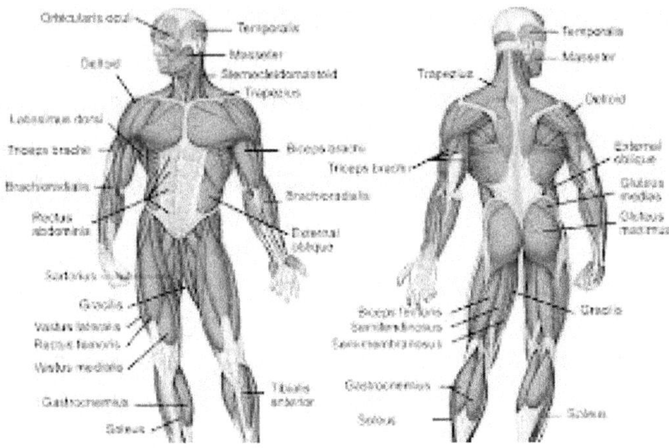

In biomechanics, such complementary opposites are termed, agonists and antagonists. For example, because high-plank scapulae (shoulder blades) are drawn onto the back (middle trapezius and rhomboids), they are pushed slightly away from the spine and flushed into the ribcage at the same time by opposing muscles (serratus anterior and pectoralis minor). These two actions allow for strength in posture, space to move into the humerus (upper arm bone) and cervical vertebrae (neck) position.

Muscle & Posture

Although this incredible activity takes place on a microscopic level, we experience the freedom of movement with less than the blink of an eye. -- The joint contains an agonist (the primary mover) and an antagonist (the opposing muscle). The body aligns with joints by coordinating its behaviour through the opposite muscles that complement it. The following are common types of posture and muscle groupings that impact posture anteriorly (to the front) and posteriorly (to the back). Rarely isolates deviation from ideal postural alignment from one region to another. For example, the forward carriage is usually the result of imbalance through the shoulders, thoracic region, low back or hips.

A chain reaction causes the whole body to have muscle imbalances. Neither is lateral and neutral rotational variability unusual. Tightness through the lower left rear, for example, will cause the left pelvis to rise. Also, rotation occurs with unilateral disparity.

In this example, the left hip may rotate forward as a result of the tight lower back muscles. Particular yoga postures can seem very difficult, or even injurious, to some forms of posture. It's often the ideal pose for a re-alignment. For example, attaining Bhujangasana (cobra posture) will be very difficult for a student with an extremely round upper back (kyphosis) and forward head carriage. Here, the instructor must remember that the practice is not about the final form of the pose, but about intent – an ideal opportunity to discover muscle support, joint and muscle mobility through the thoracic spine, chest and shoulder girdle, typically restricted areas for a kyphotic backed student. The pose will be broken down in stages.

First, seeking flexibility across the shoulder girdle chest and front, and strengthening the middle / upper back muscles. This can be simply Tadasana with hands interlaced behind the neck, extending around the arms, spreading and raising the heart, elevating the arm's bones, then pulling them down as the scapulae draw together towards the spine. By understanding common tightness or lack of mind-body connection to a particular group of muscles that may lead to misalignment, you can provide specific guidance to your students so that they can achieve greater alignment in their yoga practice and everyday life.

CREATIVE AND EFFECTIVE SEQUENCING

Sequencing Fundamentals

The series of postures that you introduce into your asana practise should be linked to your original practical or class purpose. For example, doing a high-intensity, back bending practice isn't a great way to express the intention of a tired body to regain strength. Giving a series of restorative postures, gentle twists and hip-openers would be more apt. First, set a goal for your practice or lesson and then decide which asana can help achieve that objective. At the beginning of the exercise, the body becomes firmer and more responsive. A general outline of a class provides a logical sequence to open the body's major joints systemically before attempting advanced postures. Postures may be divided into groups that are related to their anatomical body and orientation impacts. The types are of:

- Standing postures

- Hip openers

- Forward bends

- Backbends

- Twists

- Inversions

- Leg balancing

- Arm balancing

- Abdominals

- Restoratives

- Yin

Fixed and Variable Sequencing

There are several particular postures to deal with under each of the categories mentioned above. Some yoga systems such as Ashtanga Vinyasa adopt one sequence without variations. The student passes to the next sequence, or set of postures, after skillfully completing one sequence of asana.

A fixed sequence has the advantages of:

• The practitioner has a memorizable and internalize pattern to follow.

• Change can be calculated against a fixed variable — the series that is being used.

• It's better to practice by yourself in a group or with colleagues because everyone knows the rhythm.

The downsides are:

• Postures within a set series can be challenging or impossible for certain students to perform due to deficiencies in bone structure.

• Robot approach to asana practice can be generated following a set series.

• Following a set sequence does not provide an incentive for the imaginative sequence of acceptable personal practice or teaching postures.

As a new instructor or student establishing a self-practice, getting a sequence to adopt is important, and then start adding a variety of postures to match your practice and change your lessons.

Principles of Sequencing

In general, the class should begin with some form of centring and progressing through a logical sequence of postures that shift from simple to more complex and challenging. Use postures that rebalance and quiet the body and mind after class apex before Savasana.

The sequence of posture categories for a balanced class:

- Seated posture–centring

- Warm-up (simple, accessible postures or movements i.e. cat/cow)

- Downward facing dog

- Sun Salutations

- Standing postures

- Inversions (headstand or variations)

- Arm balances

- Reclining hero posture (prep for backbends)

- Backbends

- Shoulder-stand

- Twists

- Forward bends

- Savasana

To create a class using this template, sequentially transfer the list down, selecting the categories of postures that fit your class concentration that day (a pose balance, focus on back-bending, forward-bending, arm balance, etc.).

Entrainment – Centering the Class

There is a hypothesis discovered in 1666 by physicist Christian Huygens, entitled "Entraining." Essentially, the strongest energetic force within a given area would have the effect of dragging the lighter, or weaker, forces into its energy pattern. You can see one example of that in a pendulum clock. If multiple pendulum-driven clocks are put in the same space, the heavier pendulum will pull the lighter pendulums into its rhythmic pattern and give it a time to join. This idea is also at work within each group of people and is fundamental to the creation of a class environment in which true teaching can be communicated. You are in the "heaviest pendulum" spot, as the instructor. To be as bright as possible, this requires your energy: well-rested, prepared and connected to your inner teacher.

Take the time when they enter the classroom to welcome the students and make them sit comfortably, using props when necessary. Centring the class will require a brief time of meditation, wind contemplation, invocation formation or simply performing an OM. When you introduce yourself, using your intent or theme to add meaning to it, you will also have a context for the class. Stop verifying that your instructions are understood and followed when you start giving postural instructions before switching to the next pose. It will also create entrainment and provide the class with a more healthy atmosphere.

Sequencing a Mixed Level Class

All classes are very mixed, so no two students will have the same potential, energy level and physical limitations. One of the goals of a successful class is to make the class available to all students and to challenge enough for the students most capable. Using Vinyasa, transfer choices include jump-switch or step-up and-back. Using the sequence below for your self-practice. Internalize the sequence before you teach it: this will allow you to focus your attention on the students rather than trying to remember the next pose.

• Seated posture (legs crossed, half or full lotus).

• Introduce intention. Begin Ujjayi breath

• *Supta Padangustasana* (hands behind thigh)

• *Adho Mukha Svanasana* (down dog)

• *Lunge* (fingers on the floor)

• *Surya Namaskara* (3 times)

• *Trikonasana* (triangle pose)

• *Parsvakonasana* (wide angle)

• *Parsvottanasana*

- *Prasarita Padottanasana* (wide leg standing forward bend) A and C

- *Utthita Hasta Padangustasana* (hand to big toe balance)

- *Rajakapotasana prep* (king pigeon posture prep.)

- *Agnistambhasana* (double pigeon)

- *Bakasana* (crow)

- *Balasana* (child's pose)

- *Navasana* (boat) variations

- *Virasana* (hero)

- *Supta Virasana* (supine hero)

- *Ustransana* (camel)

- *Setu Bandhasana* (bridge posture)

- *Urdhva Dhanurasana* (full wheel) variations

- *Marichyasana-C* (twist)

- *Dandasana* (staff posture)

- *Upavistha Konasana* (wide leg forward bend)

- *Janu Sirsasana* (one leg forward bend)

- *Meditation/Pranayama*

- *Savasana*

Creating Intention

Before teaching set up an agenda for your students. This purpose will serve the student's highest good, and reflect your understandings in your practice and life. Intent can be practical, and affects physically, emotionally and philosophically.

The Intention of "Releasing Tension"

Physically

Choose positions and a policy that lends itself to that intent. Stress management can be enhanced by stressing steady breathing, a stable foundation, and approaching postures without provocation. Initial aim for this class to teach difficult or unfamiliar viewpoints would be contradictory.

Emotionally

Consider the emotional qualities which a release of stress creates. Qualities such as resignation, openness, lack of anxiety and resilience are measures of emotionally articulated intent.

Philosophically

The physical body affects the intellectual environment and mental body state. All three bodies are exercising and interacting with each other. Reflect on what thought attributes promote a release or lack of undue stress. These attributes can include curiosity, self-examination, seeing things with less initial judgment and a less negative and more open-hearted attitude towards others.

The art of embodying an intention when you teach a lesson is the ability to incorporate the purpose into the physical postures so that thought, feeling, and physicality resonate together and practice becomes an experience of reconnecting and revelling.

TEACHER TRAINING ON INVERSIONS

Being upside-down affects vision. Inversions facilitate circulation by manipulating blood flow through gravity. If a student has high blood pressure, a conservative approach to such inversions as the headstand should be in place. There is typically some discomfort that's linked to being upside down because it disorients at first. Encourage students to move slowly into postures like the headstand, and avoid kicking up or throwing their legs on the ground. Even the simplest of steps here can be daunting as we observe this relationship of opposite and unknown gravity. This shift in perspective and neuromuscular understanding offers an opportunity to further broaden our sense of being in the universe while reversing the effect of gravity on the body. The brain is flushed with nourishing blood, the mind is clearing, the nerves are still relaxed, and everything seems to be much more alert, giving meditation a graceful invitation.

With practice, also what's at first the hardest inversion — Salamba Sirsasana (Supported Headstand)—becomes its opposite, Tadasana (Mountain Pose), as safe, allowing students to stay in this asana for several minutes at a time. Whether in Sirsasana or Salamba Sarvangasana (Supported Shoulder Stand), students learn more complex muscle coordination that adds stability and eases several other asanas, including in fluid moves into and out of Adho Mukha Vrksasana (Handstand). The greatest physical danger in inversions is to the neck (this does not apply to Viparita Karani, the Active Reversal Pose). It is very necessary to give students clear and methodical guidance when setting up investments in such a way as to minimize this risk. It is recommended that students with cervical spine problems no longer perform any asanas which strain the neck.

Halasana (Plow Pose)

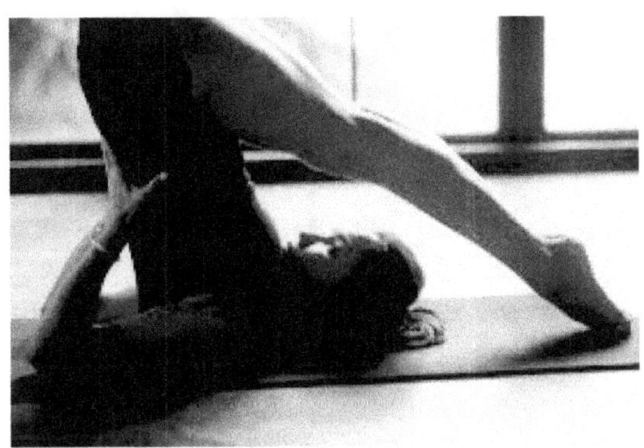

Lying supine, force the palms down and hold the feet with an exhalation over the floor (or into a block, chair, or wall). Interlace the fingers behind the back and slightly fold the shoulders underneath to add weight to the shoulders. If the neck or upper spine is under pressure, either remove one or two folded blankets under the arms and shoulders from this position or reset them. Place the feet firmly down to join and drive the thighs upwards (if necessary, pointing back), pushing the pubic bone away from the stomach to lengthen the spine. Hold arms and feet firmly planted. When spreading through the chest and moving through the spine towards the throat, bring the collarbones down. Continue upwards pushing the sitting bones, flowing around the spine.

Karnapidasana (Ear-Squeezing Pose)

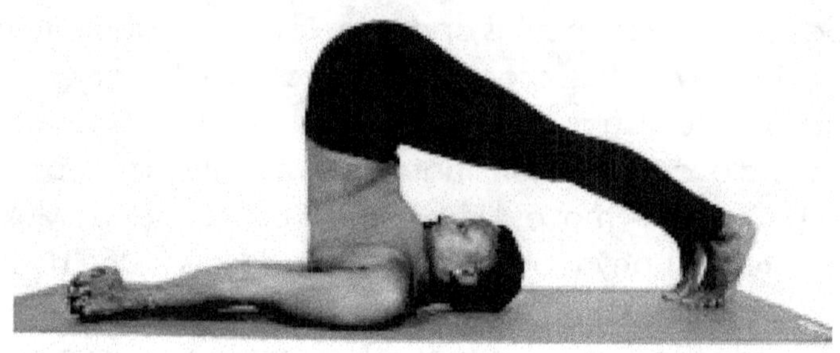

Cue Halaṣana students to lower their knees to or to the ears as they force their arms down into the ground and pull their knees into their ears while listening to the wind from the inside. Encourage you to keep your breath full and be very sensitive to excessive pressure above or below your throat.

Urdhva Padmasana (Upward Lotus Pose)

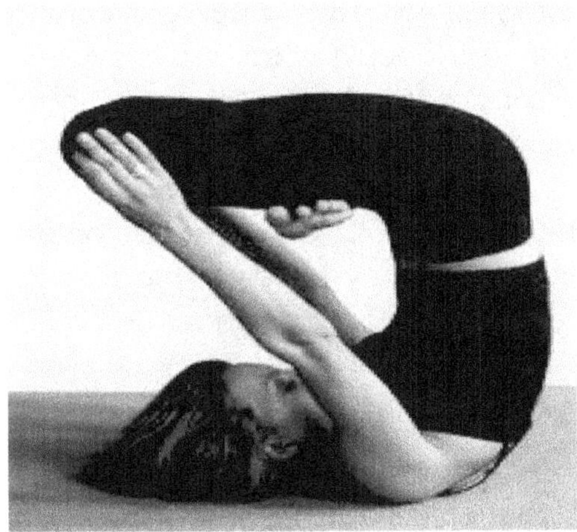

Exploring Salamba Sarvangasana (Shoulder Stand), shifting the legs to the Padmasana (Lotus Pose) posture using one hand at a time to help if needed. Stretch the lotus knees straight up, straighten the arm up and bring the knee to the hand on that side, then place the other hand and knee together. Focus on rooting muscles, spreading the throat, stretching back and retaining steadiness while breathing comfortably and spaciously. Engage bandha Mula and take a look at the nose or stomach.

INTRODUCTION TO COOPERATE YOGA

Study shows Americans spend $5.7 billion per year on yoga classes and products, including equipment, clothes, holidays, and media (DVDs, videos, books, and magazines). This statistic represents an 87 per cent increase relative to the previous study in 2004—nearly double what was previously spent. The 2008 study shows that 6.9 per cent of adults in the U.S. practise yoga, or 15.8 million. (In the previous study the amount was 16.5 million). Nearly 8% of current non-practitioners, or 18.3 million Americans, say they are very or very involved in yoga, three times the amount of research in 2004. And 4.1 per cent of non-affiliated practitioners, or around 9.4 million individuals, say they're likely to practice yoga in the coming year. The study also collected data about age, gender and other demographic factors. Yoga activities surveyed:

• 72.2% are female; 27.8% are male

• 40.6% are between the ages of 18 and 34; 41% are between the ages of 35 and 54, and 18.4% are over 55.

• 28.4% practice yoga for one year or less; 21.4% practice between one and two years; 25.6% practice between two and five years; and 24.6% practice for five years;

• 71.4% are university-educated; 27% hold postgraduate degrees

• 44 per cent of yogis have $75,000 or more in household incomes; 24 per cent have more than $100,000

The 2008 research also revealed that almost half (49.4%) of current practitioners have chosen to practice yoga to improve their overall well-being. In the 2003 study, the number was 5.6 per cent. And they continue to train for the same reason. According to the 2008 survey, 52 per cent are encouraged to practice yoga to improve their overall wellbeing. In 2003, the number was 5.2 per cent. One significant concept to arise from the study is the use of yoga as a medical treatment. According to the survey, 6.1 per cent or nearly 14 million Americans say a doctor or yoga therapist has recommended them. Also, nearly half (45 per cent) of all adults agree that yoga would be beneficial if they seek to care for a medical condition.

Questions for your Yoga business

1) What is the principal explanation given for the interest in yoga?

Canada has about 1/10 of the population in the United States In BC there are about 4 million people, many in the Lower Mainland. If the per capita estimates are the same, we either already have 15 per cent of this population practising yoga or are interested in doing it-that is 600,000 people in B.C. Density-about 200 people live in the Vancouver area, in one city block. Of the 200, that's 30 per cent. How far will a student go to your home studio walk or ride a yoga bike in? How many potential pupils are there to come?

What do you think would be the carbon footprint of a yoga studio, where the participants drive 10-15 minutes, two or three days a week each way? Is the promotion of that an acceptable business practice?

Using the demographic breakdown from the analysis above, answer as follows:

2) Where will they shop?

3) What amusements do they do?

4) How many are possibly Internet-savvy?

5) What type of clothes are they buying?

6) What kind of language would the commercial resonate with them?

7) She's fit and flexible?

8) What kind of a yoga presentation will make them feel relaxed and curious about learning more?

9) What time of day will match their yoga class schedules?

10) How many days a week do you think they want to go to yoga?

11) What would be the key deciding factor in selecting a course – price, comfort, teacher relation, class time?

12) List five excuses that would discourage anyone interested in yoga from attending a workshop or class.

13) Which per cent are beginners?

14) Courses to pre-register or drop-in?

It is a historical fact that only a very small percentage of Hindus in India were able or permitted to practice yoga. Everyone has access to yoga lessons in our society, but it appears from the above statistics that the well-to-do and educated are primarily engaged in yoga. There may be some reasons for this, but Douglas Brooks looks at the problem interestingly. He says (and I'm paraphrasing) "It takes some bourgeois complacency before one asks the question, 'Is there any more?' The challenge now is how to make the yoga practice available in a way that increases the student's selective awareness, so that they can engage in their practice in the richest way possible.

Marketing

Internet marketing, especially Google Adwords, is a very effective and inexpensive tool to promote your website to the local community – you can choose to view your advertising globally, within a province or even within a few blocks of where you're educating. Ads will appear on a request for keywords that you select, such as "Vancouver yoga studio" or "Back pain yoga."

Significant exposure can be provided in your local community through well-placed, high-quality print advertising, as well as symbiotic partnerships with massage therapists, chiropractors, natural food stores, and athletic apparel stores. Remove all obstacles between your future students and a friend in your class. Then inspire them with good teaching and a chance to engage with others within the culture. Tea after class is a great way to encourage discussion and get to know others.

YOGIC STUDY ON INSOMNIA AND FOLLOWING PRACTICE ON YOGA NIDRA

An activated nervous system occasionally causes insomnia. Postures which emphasize cooling and releasing are of great benefit to individuals suffering from this disease. So Sarvangasana (shoulder stand) and Halasana (poison-removing posture) are all right. A reasonably intense nervous energy release practice, followed by a long Savasana to encourage relaxation, is useful if the student is otherwise able to do so. Originating from the tantras, Yoga Nidra is an important method in which you consciously learn to relax. Nidra sleeping in yoga isn't seen as a relief. People feel relaxed sitting in a cosy chair with a cup of coffee, a drink or a cigarette and reading a newspaper or flipping on the TV. But this will never be enough, as a medical definition of relaxation. These are pure stimulation to the senses. True relaxation is a step above all this. For absolute relief, you must stay awake. That is Nidra Yoga, the condition of complex sleep. Yoga Nidra is a complete, systematic induction approach.

For a physical, mental and emotional relaxation. The word yoga Nidra derives from two Sanskrit words, yoga signifying union or one-pointed consciousness, and Nidra meaning sleep. During the practice of yoga Nidra, one seems to be unaware but the mind works at a deeper level of awareness. For this function, also referred to as Yoga Nidra is spiritual sleep or deep relaxation with inner consciousness. Spontaneously, contact with the subconscious and unconscious elements occurs in the transition state between sleep and wakefulness. You attain the state of relaxation in Yoga Nidra by turning inward, away from the outer experiences. If the consciousness can be separated from outer consciousness and sleep, it is very powerful and can be used in various ways, for example, to improve memory, enhance intellect and creativity, or alter one's personality.

Outline of the Practice

Yoga Nidra is a practice typically lasting 20 to 40 minutes. T here are different methods for people with hypertension and other problems, and for those who want to go deep into yoga's spiritual aspect. Yoga Nidra is an easy activity and you can learn from a recording or film. Before you start, choose a quiet space, and close the windows and doors. Switch off your radio or television, loosen your collar and tie and turn on the tape recorder. Then lie down, and listen to Shavasana's instructions. Start following the instructions, consciously. Do not concentrate, do not regulate your mind, only listen and mentally follow the instructions. The most important thing in Yoga Nidra is that you refrain from sleep. If you fall asleep you lose interest in the task you are trying to do.

Preparation for the practice

In Shavasana, Yoga Nidra has performed ed which minimizes touch sensations by eliminating contact between the limbs of the body. By turning hand palms upwards, the fingertips, which are highly sensitive touch organs, are kept away from the floor. Wear comfortable, loose clothes. Space should be neither hot nor cold and there should be no breezes or drafts aimed at the body. Visual stimuli are easily eliminated by turning the eyes off. Then the subconscious concentrates on outside sounds. If manipulation ignored all sensory stimulation then the mind would become anxious and disturb. Hence the mind is driven to think of external sounds and to move from sound to sound with the attitude of a witness. After a while, the mind loses interest in the outside world and eventually becomes silent. This way to relax the mind is called Antar Mouna. To practice Nidra yoga it prepares the mind.

Resolve

You have to pick your very own Sankalpa very carefully. The wording should be very clear and plain, otherwise, it won't penetrate the subconscious mind. A few brief statements which can be used constructively and reliably are as follows:

- I'll see my divine ability awaken.

- I'll be a constructive influence for others to develop.

- I'm going to be good with everything I do.

- I'll be more effective and more conscious.

- I'll be able to maintain optimal safety.

Just choose one Sankalpa, depending on your preferences and inclinations. Don't try to get inside. If you have selected a Sankalpa you can not move to another one. Don't expect results overnight. It takes time depending on the essence of the resolution and the degree to which it is being planted in the mind. The result depends on your sincerity and a sincerely felt commitment to fulfil your Sankalpa objective.

Rotation of consciousness

The propagation of consciousness through the different parts of the body is not an operation of meditation and involves no physical motion. During practice, there are only three conditions to be met: I rem agin alert, (ii) listening to the voice, and (iii) moving the mind very quickly in the direction provided. Repeat it mentally when the professor says 'right-hand thumb,' think of the right thumb and move on. You needn't be able to see the different parts of the body. You just have to get used to doing the same pattern, repeating the names of the different parts of the body naturally in the same way as the child learns to repeat the letters of the alphabet. You do not ask yourself what's next. The whole thing happens inside the subconscious mind.

The body parts series needs to be detailed, random and attic controlled. Some people do teach Nidra yoga very unsystematically. Sometimes they start at the shoulders and go to the toes. At times they begin with the left thumb, and at other times with the right. Hence the practice of Yoga Nidra is very formal. In Yoga Nidra, the rotation of consciousness continues in a definite sequence, beginning with the right thumb and ending with the little toe of the right foot; then the chain from the left thumb to the small toe of the left foot. Subsequent circuits continue through the heels at the back of the head, and from the head and individual facial features to the thighs.

Awareness of the breath

When these spins of consciousness have been completed, physical stimulation is then continued and completed by drawing focus to the air. In this activity one simply keeps breath knowledge; there should be no attempt to manipulate it or change it. One may watch the breath in the nostrils, in the mouth, or at the passage between navel and throat. In general, greater relaxation is achieved by counting the breaths automatically simultaneously. In addition to promoting relaxation and concentration, breath consciousness also awakens higher energies and directs them to every cell of the body. It assists pratyahara in the subtle-body activities that follow.

Feelings and sensations

Relaxation comes next to thinking and feeling plane. Feelings that are intensely physical or emotional are recalled or awoken, felt thorough and then removed. This is generally accomplished with pairs of opposing emotions like heat and cold, heaviness and lightness, pain and pleasure, satisfaction and sadness, love and hate. The mixture of feelings in Nidra yoga harmonizes the opposite brain hemispheres and helps to align our basic drives and to control normally unconscious functions. This practice also grows on the strength of the emotional plane and through catharsis leads to emotional relaxation as memories of deep feelings are relived.

Visualization

The final stage of Nidra yoga allows the mind to relax. The student visualizes the images described or listed by the teacher in this portion of the lesson. Since the often-used images have a common sense and clear connections they bring the hidden contents of the deep unconscious into the conscious mind. The practice of visualization increases the perception of oneself and relaxes the mind, purging it from disturbed or painful content. It is conducting the mind to concentrate or Dharana. Visualization progresses in advanced stages into dhyana or simple meditation.

Then, the conscious perception of the visualized object resides in the unconscious, the distinction between conscious and unconscious dissolves and the intrusive images cease to exist.

Ending the practice

The practice of visualization is usually finished with an image evoking deep feelings of peace and calmness. This indicates that the unconscious mind is highly open to new thoughts and sensations. And Nidra's yoga practice ends with a conviction. This direct order from the conscious mind to the unconscious is the seed which allows one to radically alter one's attitude, actions and destiny. It is very necessary to state the Resolution clearly and positively. This will bring a good outlook and strength of mind. One should have the true assurance that the resolution would succeed. This faith increases the effect of determination on the unconscious mind so that resolution becomes a reality in one's life. The practice of Nidra yoga is completed by gradually moving the mind from the unconscious sleep condition to the waking state.

TEACHER TRAINING PRACTICE ON FORWARD AND BACKBENDING ASANAS

Backbends:

Open body front with backbends. Gravity and natural closing of the frontal body due to posture will round the back and close the front body, both mentally, emotionally and causally (thought domain). Backbending invigorates the nervous system and can help to ease the feelings that were held. Since these postures activate the nervous system, daytime should be used for intense backbend practice, and if they are done too late at night, they can induce insomnia.

Forward bends:

These postures stretch the back of the body and close the forehead where the attention of our vision organs is on. Generally, the effects on the nervous system are more introverted, soothing and calming. The lower back should be slightly concave and the spine extended, turning the pelvic forward, before folding the torso inwards, to have a beneficial impact on an inward curve. It would be fitting for students to be sitting on a block or blanket to achieve that. Keep legs straight when standing and fold partway, helping the legs with hands-on.

Urdhva Mukha Svanasana (Upward-Facing Dog Pose)

Up Dog is an intense and powerful, awakening, back-bending Asana. Often offer the students the option of Salabhasana B as an alternative under the following conditions: lower back pain or insufficient arm, shoulder, or leg strength to hang the body on the hands and feet. First practice Salabhasana B is helpful in first learning Up Dog, which strengthens the lower back and teaches leg activation which is central in this asana. Emphasize active and balanced legs: when the legs are straight, the feet extend backwards and press down firmly, with the inner thighs spiralling upwards. Encourage the students to press their feet firmly down to create an appearance of spreading their toes straight backwards. The legs are getting more interested in rooting down the feet. From this base in the feet, instruct the students to pull their pelvis forward, away from the knees, push the tailbone back to the heels and hold the buttocks soft while allowing the pelvic weight to provide traction to the lower back. Do not advise the gluteal muscles to contract, allowing the femurs to move outside and to pinch the sacroiliac joint.

Guide the students to the full expression of asana by asking them to push their hands closely, lift their chest and establish a feeling of the focus of the backbend in their heart centre. Rooting deep into index finger knuckles helps keep controlled pressure around the hands and wrist joints, thus reducing the risk of wrist strain. Strong and balanced hand rooting also contributes to stretching the arms and raising and spreading the shoulders, which is necessary to establish the length in the spine required to enhance the backbend. The wrists are set immediately below the elbows. If the wrists are positioned in front of the shoulders, the students feel undue pressure in the lower back; the wrists will be hyperextended if they are situated further back than the shoulders. In the Chaturanga transition and backbend width where the shoulders end up relative to the wrists is determined by feet movement.

Holding the tiptoes set and rolling over them would force the hips and shoulders forward further; pulling back the feet while keeping the arms straight will result in the back of the shoulders. There's no right path forward. Rather, the unique (and varying) anatomy of each student's body — the length of their arms, legs, feet, and torso plus the degree of their back-bending arc — depends on how much to emphasize rolling over their toes versus extending their feet backwards. Proving these alternatives demonstrate the effect on the lower back, hands and overall integrity of Urdhva Mukha Svanasana. Ask students to deliberately draw the backbend curve of the spine and generate a feeling of pulling in and up the lower tips of the shoulder blades as if they were in their centre of the heart. Students with poor shoulders would appear to hang up in their arms. This tends to strain the forehead, close the heart centre, risk the breath and exacerbate the desire to dump backwards.

Encourage these students to press their hands more firmly (wrists permitting) to force the shoulders farther down and away from the ears. The head will be held at a level; the asana's final action may be to push back the head with practice, ease and relaxation. The students are encouraged to curl the palms energetically to create more space around the centre of the heart and draw the spine towards the heart to strengthen the bend while pressing the palms firmly down.

Bhekasana (Frog Pose)

Start as for Salabhasana, then put the forearms on the floor as for Naraviralasana, under the shoulders with the elbows. Explore one side at a time, first brace your right foot with your right hand and raise your right heel to the outside of your right hip. In this attempt, try to lift the elbow, and position the hand on the foot with your fingers pointing the same direction as your toes. Try to pull your right shoulder forward towards the front of the mat, square your shoulders. If flexible enough, do so with both hands and feet at the same time. Rooting the hips and bringing the tailbone down, pulling the feet into the floor while lifting the chest (being very sensitive to the knees and lower back). Try to pull the back of the shoulder blades down, lower tips of the shoulder blades moving towards the centre. Look back down, or forward, to make things simpler.

Dhanurasana (Bow Pose)

Lying out, knees bent and feet clasping back in. Flex your feet to get bandha pada activated and stabilize your knees. Rooting down through the feet, pulling on the ankles to lift the chest and legs the floor, moving the tailbone down, dragging the neck toward the heart and spreading through the collarbones. Look for the thighs to move further back to lift the chest higher, then force the feet upwards. Focus on the back curve of the middle thoracic spine. If the neck is safe then lower the head to the feet.

Eka Pada Raj Kapotasana II (One-Leg King Pigeon Pose II)

Bring the right knee straight out of Adho Mukha Svanasana's right hand and then lower the left hip and leg down to the floor. Propose as high as possible the left sitting bone to ensure (a) that the sitting bone is firmly supported, (b) that the hips are even and (c) that the inside of the right knee is not under strain. Keep the sitting bones to the ground and the hips straight, fasten the left foot with the left hand (using a brace if necessary), then draw both arms over the head to fasten the foot (or along the brace) and drop the top of the head into the foot arch. Getting the hips even and grounded in this asana is important to protect the lower back and foreknew. In the backbend, move the back leg hip forward, spiralling the leg internally to compress the sacrum to more conveniently align the back leg to pelvic. Force down the tail bone by raising the chest and pushing the elbows towards each other, generating a feeling of rising the lower tips of the shoulder blades into the heart as they rise and stretch the open heart towards the sky.

THEMING FOR THE YOGA SEQUENCE

Themeing

Every class has a heart-oriented theme, which has an essential relation to the great spiritual purposes of the asana practice. Usually, the theme focuses on cultivating a virtue — a quality of mind or heart which is a microcosmic manifestation of our Divine existence. The theme provides instructions for the attitudinal energy that infuses the poses with every breath and motion. In reality, all of the poses in Anusara Yoga are expressed from the 'inside out.' The theme is interlaced with the postural directions in the class."

One example would be "Playfulness" for a theme:

"Playfulness is seen in those who approach life with a light confident attitude. The attitude emerges from an implicit belief that we are all o.k. Basically, on a basis. We may like or dislike some of the qualities we possess but the practice of yoga allows us to see under them our true nature. Have fun with the postures as we practice today – enabling the exercise to percolate your creative side. "Playful is a mixture of terms such as play and plenitude.

There's an expansive feeling when we let go and allow ourselves a little silliness. Many concepts that require a polarity — almost opposites, including effort and retreat, unity and independence — one that yields to the other, and they work together.

Themeing a Specific Posture

If you want to add a theme to your class, it would be much more effective if you could refer to it in the context of the postures, not just at the beginning and end of the lesson.

Bakasana:

"Bend the downward dog's knees and jump slightly into your bent arms, hoping you'll land on them with your feet. Look first at this, in your mind. Unleash all irrational thinking! It is just a single phrase, a simple theme.

Writing down some synonyms that clarify your theme to keep it enjoyable for the students is a good idea: playfulness: lightness; expansiveness; without fear; with wonder; with a smile; unrestrained. Most common themes can describe the virtues of the heart and/or mind: courage, steadfastness, commitment, compassion-there are many others. If you have personal experience relevant to your subject, it can resonate with your students more profoundly than merely relating to an abstract virtue or feeling that doesn't resonate with you. There are many ways to start brainstorming about concepts – all you have to do is think about an experience you've had and how you respond to it, then discover the virtue or heart trait that was needed to manage the situation skilfully. Make it unique, and then relate it to your student's experience.

For example: "I just came back from teaching a workshop in Tofino. I was exhausted when I arrived the night before and had to drag myself to my host Natalie's regular class. I didn't feel like teaching the next morning, but after her lecture, talking to Natalie and seeing her incredible enthusiasm for the next day's workshop and all the planning she'd made to prepare something changed in me.

Let's vibrate this practice with intensity, and at the end, take a deep Savasana. 'Then, when you teach a pose, relate the virtue you spoke of – in this case, resilience – and integrate it into the postural instructions. Choose poses that go well with your theme; for example, include lots of standing poses that are held slightly longer than normal: 'From Tadasana, leap to the side of your mat, feet broad spread for Prasarita Padottanasana – broad leg forward bend. Take a deep inhalation, and feel your breath's strength pulsation as you relax your skin. Inhale your body, and bring your feet in strength. Clasp your hands behind your back as you bend your knees slightly. Knees bent, the top of your thighs press back as you fold in. Draw your tailbone on the next exhale, and return the energy reservoir through the legs and arms. Extend a little longer, with commitment. If you've got a hard time coming up with a theme you might consider:

• The hardest thing you've ever done.

• The most fun you've ever had.

• An experience that has touched you deeply.

• A time when you could have acted better, and which quality was missing at the time.

Write on each of those experiences one or two sentences, and then find the main virtue or emotion. For instance, in the sentence, "The hardest thing I've ever done was to tell my younger brother, who was 11 at the time, that our father had died," the core feeling or virtue needed was compassionate stability. Take time to write a theme for a class, share it with your group and give each other feedback. Your class theme should connect your own experience to the common experience of the school, illustrate a definition that can be expressed visually and be simple and unforgettable.

INTRODUCTION TO MEDITATION

Meditation can be overwhelming to those of us who are attracted to a physical and intense form of yoga. In a world where multitasking is the rule, the ability to sit still is an art that appears to disappear. Much of the negative behaviour we do is a response to avoiding spending time with each other or even fear. We probably fear that if we go inside we would not like what we find. The expectation is just another step towards developing a meditation practice.

We're conditioned to assume some observable benefits from research time. Progress on the journey requires both individual effort in the form of meditation and total surrender. We may not be familiar with established states of consciousness and may have no understanding of what to expect in a meditation session. Outcomes can vary. Meditation can calm the nervous system, give equanimity thinking and reduce the effects of stress. The ultimate purpose of meditation is to connect with our source, the sea of consciousness where we usually see ourselves as merely a wave, forgetting that we are indeed the ocean itself.

Just sitting

The meditation approach is simplicity at its simplest. The Zen-tradition style is spartan and concise. Only sit back. When you sit back you begin to think more about your inner world. The mind appears to move, actively operating, as opposed to the quietness of the body.

Questioning

In the questioning state, one can notice a response like aversion after a sitting time, and start questioning the source of the aversion. There's a powerful form of self-study to its source after the aversion, or whatever else happens, that proves to be quite humbling.

Dynamic meditation

This style of meditation was favoured by Osho, saying the modern mind was too focusless to do traditional sitting meditation. Interactive meditation can include gestures, free speech, nonsensical babble, music and dancing.

Nada

Nada is the sound of the universe inside us. When you close the tiny flaps of the ears with thumbs you can detect an inner ringing sound. The sound energy reveals the underlying tones, and shifts emphasis and attention to subtler layers.

All is Consciousness

The attitude is Consciousness. Note the mental movements while sitting clearly, with no effort to pause or disrupt the movements. Let the mind do what it wants, and consider it to be the work of the Supreme.

Exercise:

Take a comfortable seat so your elbows are on your feet, or just above. This will avoid painful rounding of the back, allowing you to sit away from low back pain without unnecessary pressure or disruption. Place your hands on your knees and bend your elbows so you relax. Gently shut the eyes, and let the sockets fall back. Look out for the air and note its pulsation. Only sit there for a while at the moment, anywhere from three minutes to thirty minutes, using the breath as the focus of meditation. Start with a fair period. Establish your meditation habit by finding a time and place. A place you won't be disturbed should be that room. You will find friendly and fairly quiet wherever you are. You can also create an altar where photos of loved ones or inspiring teachers can be placed on.

TEACHER TRAINING PRACTICE ON CHEST OPENING

Strap Work

(1) Hold a strap wider than the distance between your shoulder and start with your thigh strap.

(2) Inhalation by air brings the harness to heaven

(3) Exhalation by air brings the harness overhead and down to the ground

(4) Use this to raise the shoulders + stretch the thorax 5-10x

(5)This exercise is a great opportunity to do every day or to add to your practice of yoga/exercise

Puppy Pose

(1) Do this after the body has been heated or do it at 50% if the body is not warm yet

(2)Floor/block front or chin on the floor (this intensifies position)

(3) Take children to pose + prop elbows on blocks if their posture is too extreme (bend arms + tie thumbs to the neck)

(4) Focus on holding hips and breathing over your knees.

Shoulder Floor Opener

(1) Extended arm with shoulder socket MUST coordinate

(2) To ease the head to the ground or to prop up the leg.

(3)Choose to keep your back leg bent (as shown), straight or stacked over the other leg

(4)If you have gone too far and just got back off, be highly mindful

(5) Using this pose, find a long and therapeutic stretch.

Bow Pose

(1) Do this pose after warming up of the body-strengthen + opening

(2)Knees + feet start together

(3) At all times, breathe in here and know if you lose your breath (if so, go back and move slower)

(4) To make this pose, choose 30 per cent or 110 per cent – do what feels good here, focus on stretch + energy, not shape.

Wheel Pose

(1) At the end of your job, keep the mentality

(2)Modify the position of a bridge or place an additional alignment + engagement block between your thighs

(3) Like bow pose, always take a break here and note if you're losing your break and want to take back a tweaked version.

Supported Fish Pose

(1) Use two blocks to support the body-one at the second, and one at the lowest.

(2) The size of the middle block suits your ideal bra strap

(3)Take this pose to ground up at the beginning of your yoga practice or to screen your yoga practice

(4)Wave the stance into the sequences yin/restore

(5) Do this every day to fight for your moving lifestyle.

TEACHER TRAINING PRACTICE ON ELBOW, WRIST AND UPPER BODY

The elbow and wrist are closely related in terms of both the joint dynamics and soft-tissue structures. The elbow joint is an ingenious structure that functions as a hinge but also provides stability in rotation. It is composed of 3 joints. The articulations between the humerus and ulna, and the humerus and radius allow flexing and stretching. The articulation between the radius and ulna allows for supination and pronation; it is a rotation of the radius inside the annulus ligament.

The structure of the bones intersecting at the elbow joint provides support for the elbow. The valgus is a normal deflection at the elbow joint. This is usually higher in females than in males. To stabilize it we recommend relaxing slightly from a full extension or using a belt around the elbows in weight-bearing exercises. Both help strengthens the flexor and extender muscles which act on the elbow joint in a balanced manner. "The wrist is a very fragile organ which needs mobility but stability." The carpal bones allow for a wide range of hand movements and abilities in all their articulations.

How many useful and beautiful things human hands have made, how many hands can interact and how much hands are required for touch and communication. Exercises in Indian dance for the hands have developed into sophisticated art. The exercises in this chapter aim to maintain or improve the hands' functions, to give them enough mobility, but also to learn to use the arms, hands and finger muscles in a balanced way. This is particularly important because muscles do not support the wrist: there is no link between any of the ten tendons around the wrist and any of the carpal bones. If a patient has fallen on the extended wrist and has constant pain the wrist should be tested for possible fracture of the carpal bones.

Exercise: Shake hands

Aims: *mobilizing and relaxing the wrist and hand.*

1. Sit on the floor straight, or in a chair.

2. Bend your right elbow over your abdomen so your right hand is above it.

3. Place the right wrist with the left hand underneath and shake hand for 3–5 breaths at a regular pace; the right hand is inactive.

4. Grips the small finger side of the right hand with your left hand and shake the right hand for 3–5 breaths at a regular pace; the right-hand remains inert.

5. Check points 2–4 for the left-hand check.

Refined work

• Retain different parts of the wrist to meet the various parts of the joint.

• Keep various parts of the hand side of the little finger to touch different areas of the hand.

Exercise: Wrist circumduction

Aim: To get the wrist joint primed.

1. Sit on the floor straight, or in a chair.

2. Sit on your right ribs, with your right hand in front and away from your belly, your upper right arm and elbow.

3. Clog both the right and left fingers together.

4. Place your right elbow on your right ribs and make circular motions for 3–5 breaths with your right hand while keeping the right lower arm height; make the motions smooth and round.

5. Replay points 2–4 for the left forearm.

6. Finish sitting for a few minutes, with your hands behind you, resting on your thighs.

Exercise: Carpal tunnel stretch

Goal: Carpal tunnel stretching.

1. Sit on the floor straight, or in a chair.

2. Place your right elbow with your hand facing your abdomen and the palm facing upwards on your right ribs.

3. Keep your left hand on your right hand, your thumb on the back of your hand to stretch it

4. Hold for 3–5 breaths and then release gently.

5. Place your left thumb on the back of your right wrist and repeat points 3 and 4 to make wrist extension and carpal tunnel stretch more effective.

6. Relax 2–3 hand-held breaths.

7. Repeat points 2–6 for the left side.

TEACHER TRAINING PRACTICE ON LOWER BACK

Exercise: Baby back-bends

Aims: *mobilizing the lumbar spine into back-bending, strengthening and relaxing the lumbar area.*

1. Lie comfortably on your back, with your arms facing the ceiling above your chest and palms; use a folded blanket under your abdomen when you need gentle support for your hip bones; cover your forehead with a small pillow or folded towel so your nose is free and your neck relaxes.

2. Slightly draw the lower abdomen inwards, so gently that you can resume your regular breathing.

3. Feel the groins digging into the ground.

4. Keep your lower abdomen slightly compressed, lift your right leg with an exhalation; your knee is straight and your foot is in dorsiflexion.

5. Hold for 2–3 breaths; when easing the mild contraction of the lower abdomen, lower the leg so that you can get this movement again.

6. Bring down your leg with an exhalation; feel the relief in the lumbar region, and relax your abdomen.

7. Relax and take 1–2 breaths.

8. Repeat points 2–7 on the left leg.

9. Perform the whole cycle up to 5 times but only as long as you can breathe naturally.

10. Stretch your right arm above your head after the last go; raise your left hand, turn right with your right arm under your chin; bend both knees; stay comfortably lying on this side for a few breaths. As you push your left hand up to a seated position, let your left foot fly freely away from you. If you choose to start from the left side, move to your left side the same way.

Stronger variations

a. Repeat 1–7, except for simultaneous raising of both legs. You should place your hands flat under your forehead's hip bones.

b. Both knees bend, feet in dorsiflexion; repeat points 2–7, when raising both legs bent. If this action is performed correctly, the knees don't move far from the floor.

Workout: Hold four roots

Goals: Reinforce lumbar spine, balance.

1. Start with a modified kneeling position; knees and feet are joined together, elbows bent, elbows under the shoulder joints, and lower arms parallel. When appropriate, rest your elbows on a folded blanket.

2. Stretch backwards one leg at a time, knees away from the floor; only the toes meet the floor; hands, feet, and head are in a line.

3. Keep your buttocks straight, and slightly suck your lower abdomen in.

4. Rest for 1–3 breaths.

5. Keep your elbows and shoulders the same, knee down to the floor, one at a time. If your hands shift closer together, wear a brick or book in place.

6. Perform points 2–5 3–5 times; change the order in which you move backwards on the left and right side for repetitions, and the order in which you lower your knees at the end.

7. To end your stay in the balanced four-point kneeling position for a few breaths; place your buttocks on your heels or a folded pillow and relax for a few breaths.

Stronger variation

1. Start as indicated in points 1–3,

2. Maintaining the neutral lumbopelvic role by safe buttocks and abdominal muscle activity, simply lift the right leg as long as the hips stay at the same level and no rotation occurs

3. Rest for 1–3 breaths.

4. Return to Start Place (reference 1).

5. Rising your left leg as described in points 2 and 3 then returning to the modified four-point kneeling starting position.

6. Do points 2–5 3–5 times.

7. To finish, return to the modified four-point kneeling position; place your buttocks on your heels or a folded blanket, and relax for a few breaths.

TEACHER TRAINING PRACTICE ON PAVANAMUKTA ASANA

In the yoga system, the concept of asanas begins with the Pawanmuktasana series. The key idea behind these asanas is to provide flexibility in areas of the body joints. We can't practice such asanas properly without allowing adequate flexibility in joints. Pawanamuktasana is the best technique for stretching joints. This asana is important for those people who strive to do something wonderful in the area of higher stages of yoga. You can not go up to higher levels for asanas without proper practise of this asana. The proper practise of this asana provides flexibility in the joints and decreases muscular rigidity. It can not be ignored this asana, as the subconscious effect of this basic and natural practice affects the entire body and mind. Etymologically this term-pawanmuktasana means three aspects which are Bawana namely air, wind or necessary breath, Mukta is free and asana means sitting posture; hence, it is a yoga posture from which the stagnant air of the body joints is removed.

Those stagnant airs are the reason behind arthritis. The practice of this asana also has a positive and subtle impact on heart attacks and high blood pressure. The best thing is one can do this no matter what age criteria. This is now being taught in these days as naturopathy and has become a standard part of modern medicine.

Following is the primary position of Pawanmuktasana:

· Sit straight on the concrete, keeping both the knees and feet together

· Hold neck and vertebra in the same place

· Put your palms on the floor or cover with your stomach, keep your fingers outstretched

· Press the palm to hold the trunk straight, while the neck bends backwards

· Close your eyes now and deliberately breathe

· Get physically ready for work

· Keep on running with your eyes open

· Keep a good respiratory balance still

· Eventually return to the primary position

· Be conscious of the affected limbs and the changes that can occur there.

Toe Bending (Padangulin Naman)

Pangolin Naman is an Indian translation for Toe Bending pose. You can learn this asana as below:

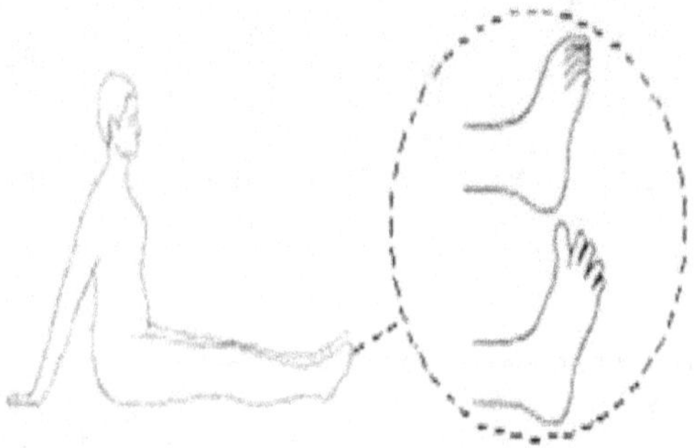

Routine:

· Give yourself the prime role.

· Split the legs while maintaining some space.

· Foot emphasis.

· Inhale deeply and move the toes quickly backwards.

· Exhale, as the feet move.

· Be mindful of foot pressure. Do not change ankle.

· Keep your eyes closed while you exercise.

· Initially repeat the exercise for 10 times.

· Open your eyes after work out.

Respiratory pattern:

· Inhale deeply as your feet are spinning.

· Exhale your toes as they move.

Consciousness:

· On respiration.

· Abstract numbers.

Ankle Bending (Gulf Naman)

Gulf Naman is an Indian translation for Ankle Bending pose. You can learn this asana as below:

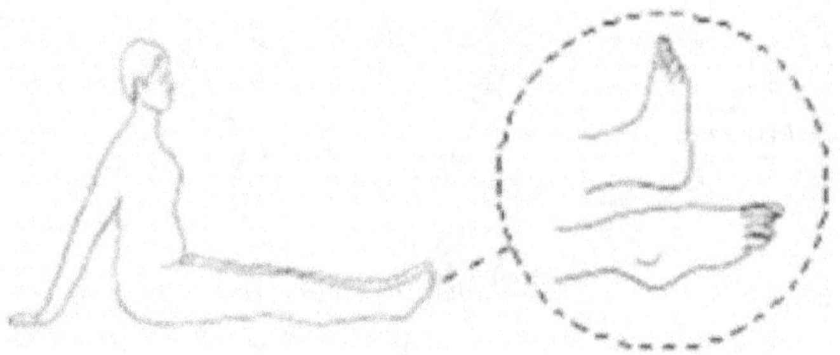

Routine:

· Get into position at the foundation.

· Split the legs while maintaining some space.

· Put ankles on.

· Let it touch the surface of the heel.

· Inhale deeply as feet are spinning.

· Exhale as you step forward on your feet.

· Stretch the toes outwards.

· Close your eyes during the exercise.

· Emphasis on moving anchor.

· If necessary, switch the ankles back and forth for a while.

· Have the exercise repeated 10 times.

Note: Don't lift your leg to a level above. Do it maintaining contact with the surface.

Respiratory pattern:

· Inhale as feet is spinning.

· Exhale the feet as they move.

Consciousness:

· On respiration.

· Abstract numbers.

· Extended foot, knee, calf and leg muscles, or joint.

Ankle Rotation (Gulf Chakra)

Gulf Chakra is an Indian translation for Ankle Rotation pose. You can learn this asana as below:

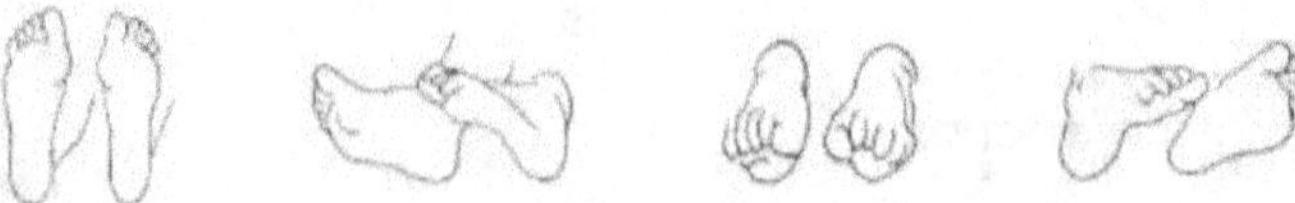

Routine:

· Train yourself first.

· Set the legs apart, both straight and short.

· Turn the feet in the direction of the clockwise and anti-clockwise direction, and the heels contact the floor.

· Emphasis on moving the body, in the right direction or not.

· Move your foot concurrently or separately if you can't do it at once.

· Keep your ankles on the watch.

· Breathing Regular and Steady.

· Repeat for 10 times and then bring the legs together.

· Rotate the ankles ten times-first in direction of the clockwise direction and then in direction anti-clockwise.

· Tie toes together.

· Do not cause the knees to elevate.

· Keep the body just and straight.

· Do it too with eyes closed.

· Keep vigilant for respiratory patterns.

· Close your eyes and brace for the next session of work.

Respiratory pattern:

· Inhale upward motion.

· Breathe out a turn downwards.

Consciousness:

· On respiration.

· Abstract numbers.

· Spinning.

Ankle Crank (Gulf Ghurnan)

Gulf Ghurnan is an Indian translation for Ankle Crank pose. You can learn this asana as below:

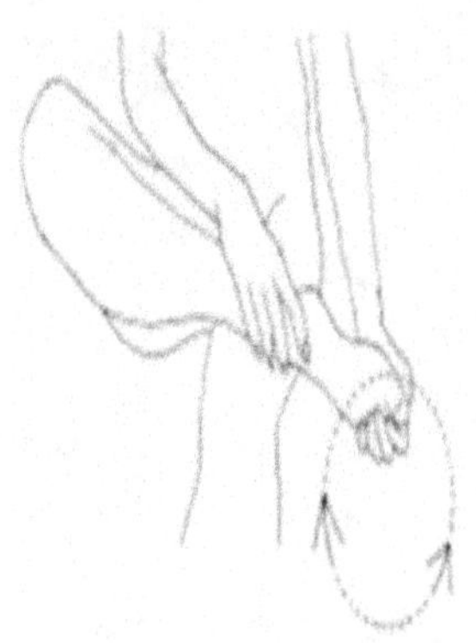

Routine:

· No change in Primary Position.

· Hold the spinal cord and neck in the same place.

· Standard is eye-opening with ease.

· Bend the right knee to the left leg, then place the sole on.

· The foot shall protrude outwards.

· Hold the right foot to the right.

· Fasten left-hand toes to the right foot.

· Steadily rotate the right foot in clockwise and anti-clockwise direction ten times with the aid of the left hand.

· Perform this exercise with the left leg positioned on the right thigh.

· The joints in the ankle remain alert.

· Breathe rhythmically with rotation.

· Note the soothing feeling of a closed-eye ankle joint.

· Return to first place until the exercise is done.

· Keep your eyes closed, and have fun.

· Close your eyes to the next series of activities and prepare yourself.

Respiratory pattern:

· Breathe in upward during the move.

· Exhale during step-down.

Consciousness:

. On the air.

· Abstract numbers.

· Rotation.

Benefits:

· Allow the return of depleted lymph and venous blood;

· Lighten the cramping and weariness.

· Prevent venous thrombosis, particularly in patients bedridden following surgery.

Kneecap Contraction (Januphalak Akarshan)

Januphalak Akarshan is an Indian translation for Kneecap Contraction pose. You can learn this asana as below:

Routine:

· Be the first to linger.

· Contract the muscle around your right knee and then move your kneecap down to your shoulder.

· Contract within 3 to 5 seconds.

· Release the contraction and return the kneecap to normal.

· Do 5 times.

· Repeat this even with left kneecap five times.

· Then figure it out on both kneecaps.

Respiratory pattern:

· Inhale and hold your breath as your contract.

· Relax the knee muscles while exhaling.

Consciousness:

· On respiratory pattern.

· Abstract numbers.

· The uproar.

Knee Bending (Janu Naman)

Janu Naman is an Indian translation for Knee Bending pose. You can learn this asana as below:

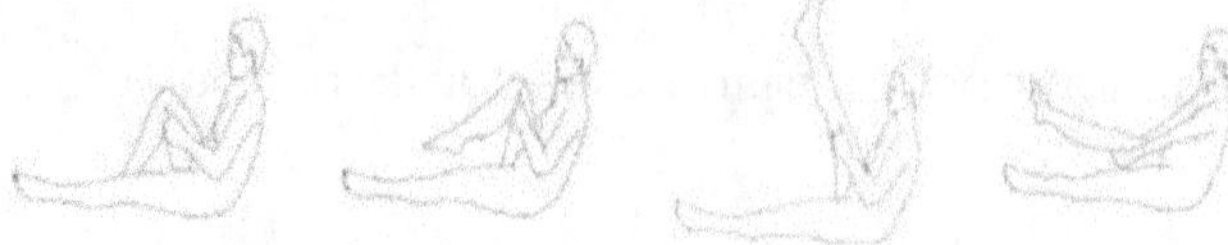

Routine:

· Body aligns in the primary position.

· Bend the knee and bring the sole off the surface.

· Thumbs cut behind the elbows.

· Raise your knees to shoulder level and keep your feet down.

· Keep the arm as straight as you can, thus bending the elbow.

· Ensure a healthy neck and spinal cord.

· Inhale as the legs straighten, slowly and deeply.

· Do not allow a heel or the toes to hit the floor.

· Thighs will rise to chest level as you exhale.

· Hold left leg straight.

· Instead do it on both hands 10 times.

· Keep your respiration pattern and thighs primed.

· Apply more thigh pressure to your abdomen as you exhale, and lift your thighs to your chest.

· Bring both legs back into the basic position following completion of the exercise.

Contraindications:

· High Blood pressure.

· Heart patients.

TEACHER TRAINING ON SEATED ASANA

Supta Parivartanasana (Reclined Revolved Pose)

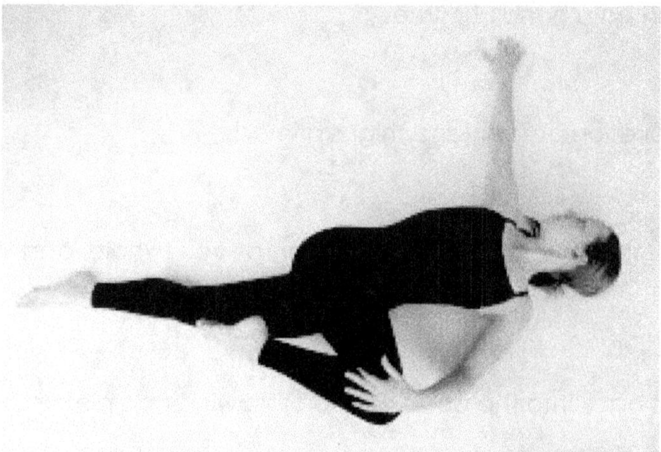

Lie supine, knees in toward the mouth as in Apanasana (Wind-Relieving Pose), arms out, palms down. Looking over, take the leg off to the left. Alternatively, keep the left leg straight onto the floor and push forward the right knee. The bent-knee position is clearer on the lower back. Enable students to be more interested in keeping their shoulder on the floor in the twist held than in getting the knee to the floor, thereby twisting the thoracic spine and not the lower back. Place the shoulders and palms firmly in core exercise while moving the hands, inhale over the elbows, exhale back to the middle.

Bharadvajrasana B (Sage Bharadvaj's Pose B or Simple Noose Pose B)

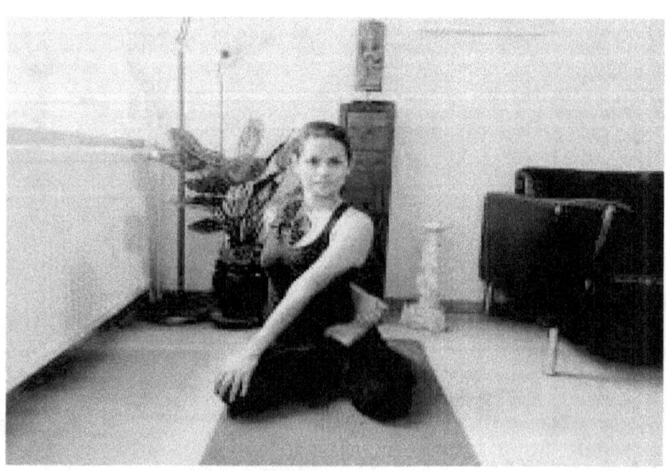

Be very aware of knees, and proceed with caution. Start as for Bharadvajrasana A except in positioning Virasana to draw the right heel close to the right hip and draw the left foot into half lotus. Twisting to the left, move the left hand behind the back and catch a piece of fabric, the right inner thigh or the lotus foot while catching the right leg. Try putting the left palm on the floor under the left knee and pointing to the left foot. The sitting bones are grounded, with each inhalation the spine becomes elongated, using hand clasps to control the twist at each exhalation. Develop a sensation of pushing the upper spine into the centre of the neck, dragging the blades down the back of the shoulder and spreading the collarbones. Turn the head to the right and draw the chin down slightly towards the right side, turning the torso to the left.

RESTORATIVE YOGA

Restorative yoga is a type of Yoga practice which is deeply relaxing. It is a receptive and not aggressive operation. There are five to twenty minutes of restorative yoga poses unlike the more intense styles of yoga which pose "flow" through each other. During this time, you are held in "shapes" when covered with boards, blocks or bolsters (pillows). The shapes resemble the forms of some more violent poses found in Ashtanga, Vinyasa, or Iyengar, such as a rear bent, forward bend, twist, or inversion. When you're in the poses you're completely assisted in a specific position that helps you attain the desired benefit — it may expand your lungs, alleviate stress in your lower back, or any of the other benefits, as well as make you feel healthy enough to "let go."

Simple Neck Stretches: Allow the head to fall forward and relax around any area that maintains tension for one to three full breaths, and then return to centre. Enable the head to fall back on an exhalation, open the throat; lift the head on inhalation towards the centre. (If the student is sitting next to the wall, let them drive their heads against the wall. If they can touch the wall with their heads, they will relax their heads against the wall; if they can not reach the wall, they can go as far as they can comfortably.)

Quick Shoulder Rolls: Roll up, back and around the shoulders, alternating movement with the wind. Inhale and take the head up to the ears; exhale, takedown and round the neck down. In the same direction, inhale, take your shoulders back and up; exhale, lower them to and fro.

Torso Circles: Sitting in a cross-legged stance, holding hands on the knees and keeping the torso straight, moving the torso in one direction from the hips and then in the other.

Upavista Konasana, Baddha Konasana, Dandasana Combo: open the legs to Upavista Konasana (Seated Wide Angle Pose) and extend the legs, push down the knees and through the feet, keep the legs bound. Stretch, and point the feet together, alternately. Place the hands in the prayer position and move the feet together, bring the feet to Baddha Konasana (Cobbler's Pose), then extend the feet to Dandasana (Staff Pose) with the hands remaining in the prayer position. Place your hands slightly behind the pelvis, raise the sternum, place your shoulder blades on your back, gently draw your shoulder blades parallel to each other, and lengthen your spine. Depending on your students and time you can explore these asanas further as part of your warm-up series. For students with limited mobility, stamina or strength, the hands should remain on the floor to help move between the postures.

Cat-Cow in table position on all fours: legs hip-width apart with hands and elbows on the surface, spin upward, inhale and exhale downward. Start coordinating the motion of air. Then move the spine from side to side, keeping the legs perpendicular to the floor and turning the shoulder and pelvis towards each other from side to side and turning the head around to look at the hip on either side. Exhale while turning your head and hips toward each other as you reach the middle. Go back to the Centre. The hips may also be rotated pausing for one or two seconds in both directions, where any sensations are maintained and comfortable.

Adho Mukha Svanasana (Downward-Facing Dog): take the buttocks back to the heels from the table position and spread the arms over the floor; put the hands on the floor without bringing them under your shoulders and return to the table position and extend the legs as you raise the coccyx to the sky. Place the knees down to the wall behind you, relax, lower one heel towards the floor and lift the other leg at the knee. Drop the heels towards the floor and lift the feet to make the students more flexible.

Add or delete any stance that will more completely help your students. Now you can step through your series of restorations.

TECHNIQUES ON STANDING VARIATIONS

Standing asanas forms the important physical foundation for asana in general practice. Students on their feet begin to understand how a solid foundation gives support through their hands, pelvis, spine, arms and head. They also discover a solid foundation is sturdy, beginning with the activation of pada bandha in the feet. Blending sthira and sukham in the standing asanas, the students begin to find samasthihi (equal standing), which invokes a consciousness of attitude and equanimity as they experience the bond between the body, air, mind and spirit. By reinforcing this sense of equanimity, students gain an inherent understanding of how the lightness of focusing on being grounded enables them to go about their yoga practice and daily life with greater ease and joy.

Standing asanas are categorized into three categories : (1) spun females outside, (2) spun females neutrally or internally, and (3) standing asanas. Externally rotated standing asanas tend to stretch the inner groin and thighs while stressing the outside rotors and abductors. In general, standing asanas which are rotated internally strengthen adductors and internal rotators while stretching external rotators and abductors. (Neutral rotation in its action and impact is similar to internal rotation, but the rotational effort is very slight.) Standing asanas strengthen the entire standing leg and pelvic girdle while offering an opportunity to examine the instinctual fear of falling while moving into steadier balance.

Padangusthasana (Big Toe Pose)

For Padangusthasana, fold forward with pada bandha in both feet as for Uttanasana, then grab and pull up on the big toes while extending the chest forward as for Ardha Uttanasana; then fold down, force the elbows away from each other and spread the shoulder blades down the neck. Start for Uttanasana as you can. Radiate down through the legs to firmly base the feet and stimulate the thighs; rotate the femurs internally, pitch the pubic bone back and forward, and stretch the sternum towards the floor. Try to bear the weight on while the heels are grounded. Lengthen the spine by the weight and movement of the body.

Malasana (Garland Pose)

Cue and demonstrate verbally from Tadasana, separating the feet slightly wider than the hip distance and then gradually lowering the knees until they are fully squatted (if necessary use a chair or block against a wall).

Anjaneyasana (Low Lunge Pose)

In stepping back the right foot and lowering the knee down to the floor for Anjaneyasana, emphasize maintaining the length of the spine and the flexibility of the heart centre. Students whose knees are sensitive to pressure, when placing on the floor, will place padding under the grounded knee Consider providing the following instructions to help break down and integrate the various habits in this asana: partially straighten the front leg, put the hands on the thighs, and develop a slight rear pelvic tilt to maintain pelvic neutrality. Gradually raise the front knee to intensify the lung and the hip flexor stretch, thus preserving pelvic neutrality. Play with slowly moving in and out of the full range of the lung, eventually releasing into a deeper stretch in the hips and groin.

Ask students to lower their arms by their hands until completed in the lunge, turn their palms out to move their arms outward, and then lift overhead. Ask the students to look down with their arms overhead for a moment and soften their lower front ribs inward while maintaining pelvic neutrality, then attempt to move their arms backwards without letting their lower front ribs protrude. You should keep the arms away from the shoulders, and hold the head straight. Invite students who, while raising across their sides, chest, back, arms and fingertips, should keep their elbows straight to press their palms overhead together. Look at the eyes, if the neck is good.

Ashta Chandrasana (High Lunge Pose or Crescent Pose)

From Tadasana, instruct students to step back from their left foot for about four feet, or, instead, from Adho Mukha Svanasana, ask students to step up their right foot next to their right hand, then draw their hands to their hips while pressing straight on the front knee. Cue students to use their hands to brace the pelvic level while firmly pushing back through the raised back heel, then keep the pelvic level and the rear leg engaged while bending the front knee straight into the line above (not beyond) the head. Alternatively extending and flexing the front knee encourages displacement of the hip flexors. Then encourage the students to lower their arms by their knees, turn the palms out and move the arms outward, then stretch the arms out and up overhead, either break the shoulder gap or press the palms together while either looking forward or at the tips of the thumb, whether they can keep their elbows fully extended.

TEACHER TRAINING PRACTICE ON THEME CLASS

The measures in learning and practice must be small enough to follow, to sustain enthusiasm and to avoid injury. In comparison, the effects of the experiment should be observed, understood and convincing. This means careful preparation is needed because asanas are more complex activities. Primary steps must be learned first before transitioning to more complex asanas or new positions. For certain asanas, most basic exercises are sufficient preparation.

You should choose the best basic training activities based on the specific area and goals you need to focus on. Among the asanas, the standing poses are good practice for most other asanas and are recommended for beginners. You should apply asanas and forward bends next to the sitting, and then the twists. Only then would there be a question about reversals and backbends. In Salamba Sīr asana and Salamba Sarva asana, the basic prerequisites for learning these Asanas are addressed. The use of props helps us to learn about these asanas and to improve their precision. With can practice progressively the props can be reduced. A balanced system covers all types of motion. Any route should be logically designed and built up slowly.

This especially applies to the directions where movement can be restricted. The routes and the phases of motion should not be mixed; there should be no "jumping" between different directions. When doing asymmetric asanas, there should be a centric, symmetric location between and at the end. Every plan, soothing and calming, should complete.

For particular emphasis, there are many ways to build a program:

• Sequences with a vibrant, radiant accent. This may be a combination of fast-paced standing poses, or twists and back-bends. There are cycles of Jumping.

• Movements relaxing and recuperating (Resting poses to prepare pra ayama).

• Sequences based on one group of asanas, for example, some standing asanas prepared with some simple exercises, finished with forward-bending asanas and relaxation.

• Use the basic exercises and asanas to focus on a specific part of the body.

• Implement a general plan which covers the whole body.

Examples of sensible mixtures are:

• standing and sitting asanas

• standing asanas and inversions

• forward bendings and twists

• backward bendings and twists

• forward bendings and inversions.

It is recommended that you begin and spend a few minutes sitting to prepare your mind for the practice and end with relaxation. Collecting basic asanas training exercises is directly a result of the exercise's condition and objectives. These suggestions offer various possibilities for combining simple exercises with asanas well suited to the situation. If the study is focused on a thorough diagnosis and medical assessment and applied with caution, work with good results is very likely to be enjoyable.

Some examples of how to apply such criteria are as follows:

1. The backstretch of the legs may be prepared for Parsvottanasana via the changed Supta Pada Hasana.

2. It is necessary, through exercise, to prepare the consciousness and strength of the feet arches for all standing poses.

3. It is possible to prepare the backstretch of the legs by revised Supta Pada gu hasana for Adho Mukha Svanasana and all other Asanas with emphasis on stretching the legs.

4. We may learn by exercise to be conscious of the hands.

5. For Adho Mukha Svanasana and Adho Mukha V k asana, the four-point kneeling variants prepare the elbow power.

REFERENCES

1. Pranayama, Kriyas, Bandhas, Nadis
2. Anatomy of Hatha Yoga_ A Manual for Students, Teachers, and Practitioners

3. Asana, Pranayama, Mudra and Bandha

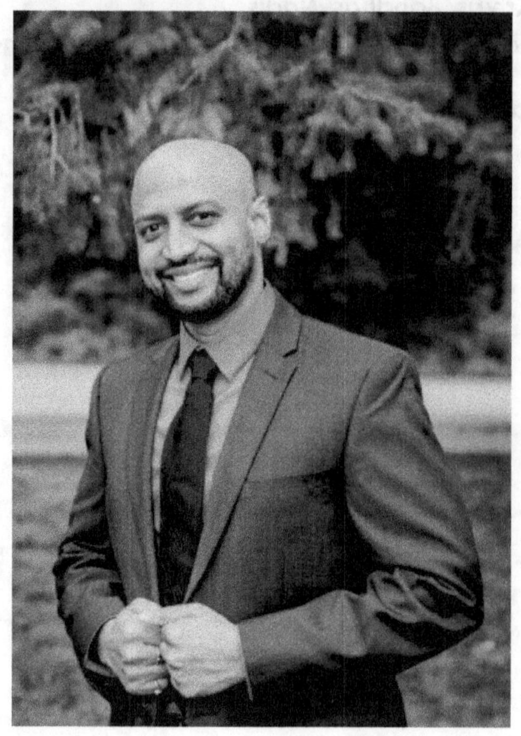

Dr. Sriram Ananthan

https://sriramananthan.com

Here are lists of Dr. Sriram Ananthan books

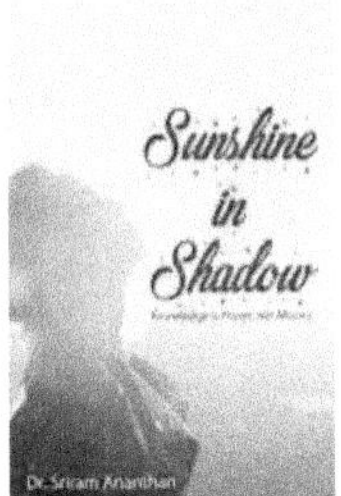
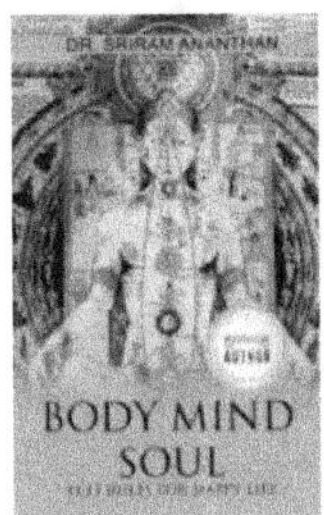

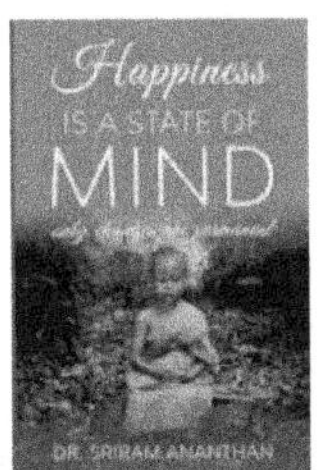
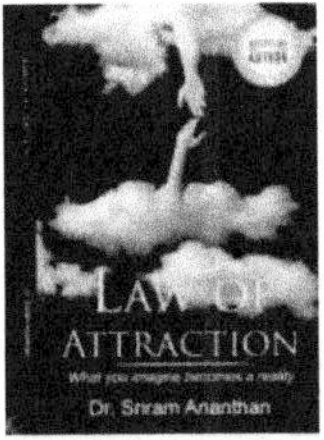

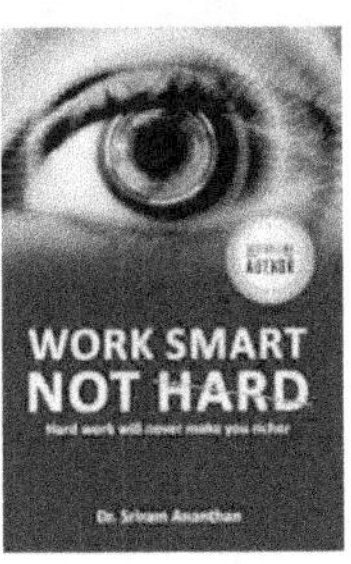
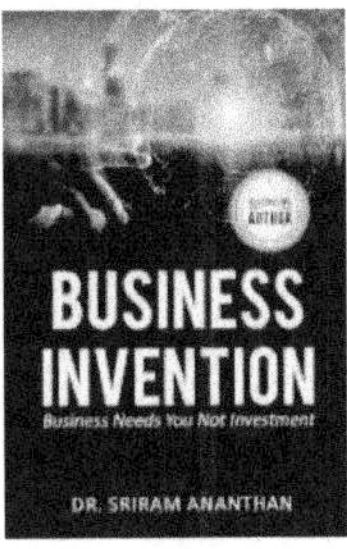